## 1st International Congress on World Food Policy: Policy Realignment in Response to Global Challenges

*Coordinated by Alfonso Sánchez-Carrasco*

# Book *of* Abstracts

Westphalia Press
An Imprint of the Policy Studies Organization
Washington, DC

Book of Abstracts



Westphalia Press
An imprint of Policy Studies Organization
1367 Connecticut Avenue NW
Washington, D.C. 20036
info@ipsonet.org

ISBN: 978-1-63723-551-5

Daniel Gutierrez-Sandoval, Executive Director
PSO and Westphalia Press

Updated material and comments on this edition
can be found at the Westphalia Press website:
www.westphaliapress.org

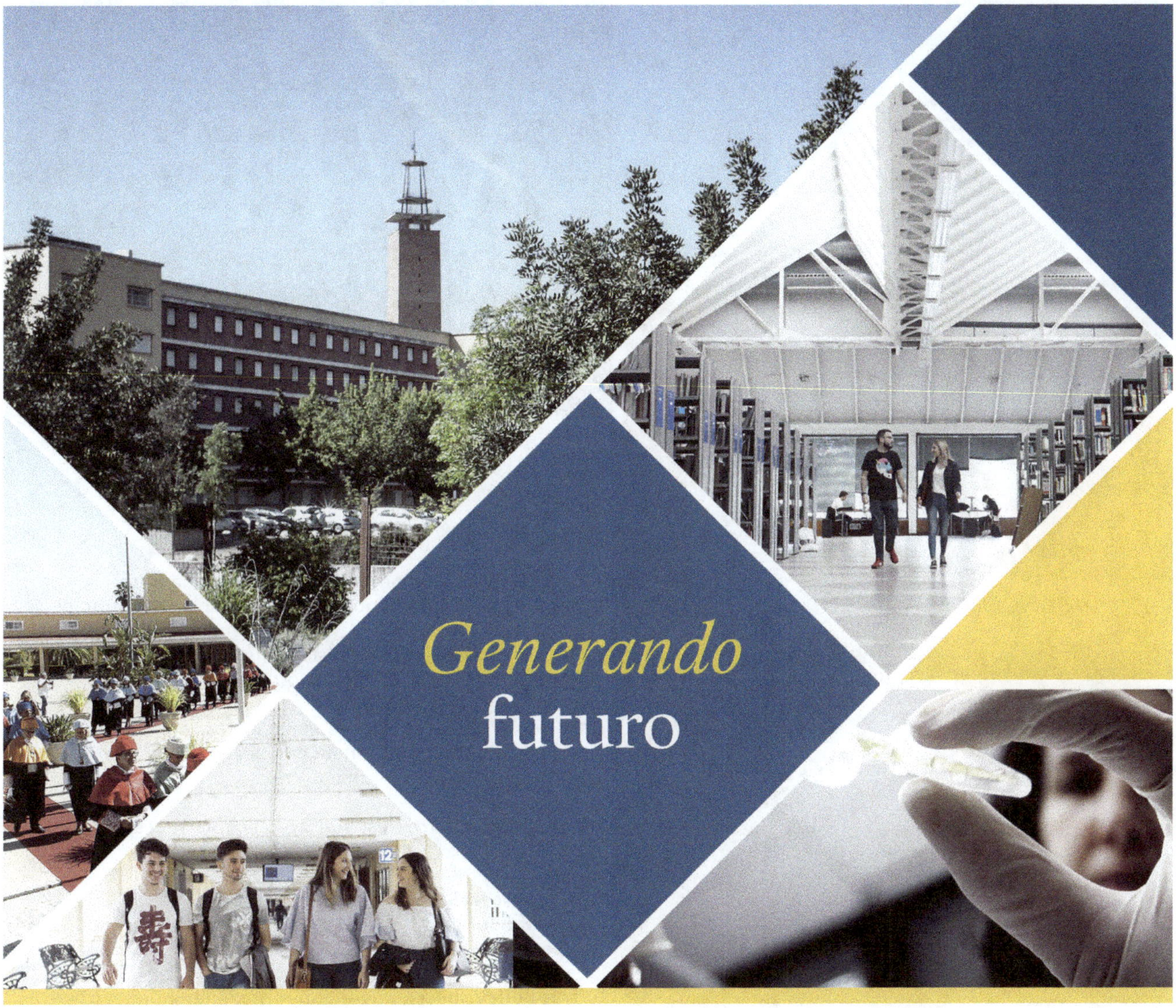


UNIVERSIDAD PABLO DE OLAVIDE SEVILLA

UNIVERSIDAD PABLO DE OLAVIDE 20 Aniversario CIENCIA POLÍTICA Y DE LA ADMINISTRACIÓN

# 20 años del Área de Ciencia Política y de la Administración en la Universidad Pablo de Olavide

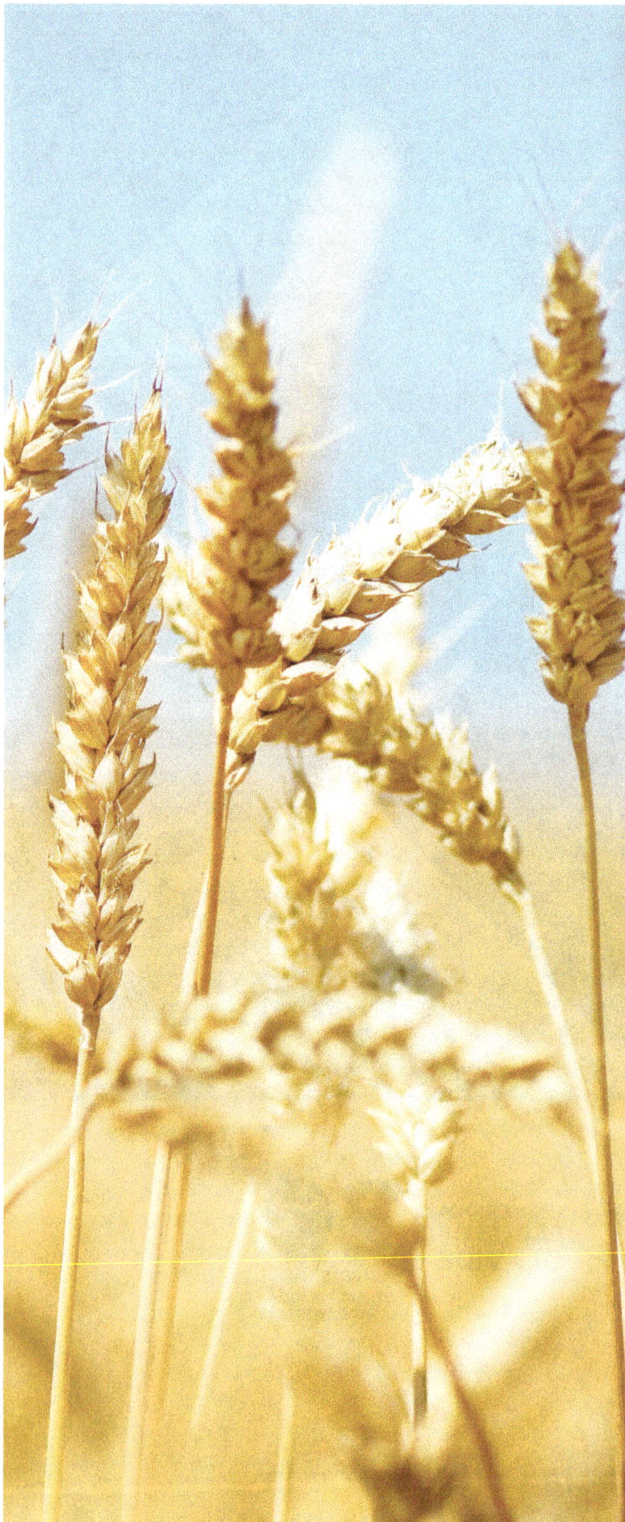

# WFP

## WORLD FOOD POLICY

VOL 12. NO. 2 NOVEMBER 2026

World Food Policy (WFP) is a biannual multidisciplinary journal covering scholarly articles on food (in)security. WFP is intended for students, academics specialists, general readers and practitioners on the field.

Provided that articles make a clear and explicit contribution to the field, we accept three types of manuscripts:

**1. Research articles:** address a scholarly research problem.

**2. Research notes:** examine issues of methodological or ethical importance within food security studies.

**3. Policy shorts:** cover issues of contemporary interest and significance to food policy.

For more information: https://onlinelibrary.wiley.com/journal/23728639

PSO

# About the Policy Studies Organization

The Policy Studies Organization (PSO) is a publisher of academic journals and books, sponsor of conferences, and producer of programs. It seeks to disseminate scholarship and information to serve those making and evaluating policy. It was founded to serve those in a variety of fields who were interested in how public policy and organizational policy were being studied and discussed.

The PSO includes senior executives, undergraduate and graduate students, state legislators, architects, judges, military officers, environmentalists who want to "green" decision making, NGO executives who worry about the future of volunteerism, professors who are working on curriculum revision, government officials in numerous agencies — in short, PSO is for intellectually active people of all persuasions.

For more information: ipsonet.org

PSO

1527 New Hampshire Ave NW
Washington, DC 20036

**How to cite the book:**

World Food Policy. (2026). Book of abstracts: 1st International Congress on World Food Policy (Seville, Spain, May 8-9, 2026). Westphalia Press.

https://westphaliapress.org/2026/07/28/book-of-abstracts-first-international-congress-on-world-food-policy/

**How to cite a specific abstract:**

example (APA 7th edition):

Echanove, J. (2026). Strengthening food governance through the right to food: Human rights-based approaches for resilient and inclusive agrifood systems. In World Food Policy: Book of abstracts, 1st International Congress on World Food Policy (pp. 1-2). Westphalia Press.

https://westphaliapress.org/2026/07/28/book-of-abstracts-first-international-congress-on-world-food-policy/

# Index

# Welcome Letter

In 2026, we will host the 1st International Congress on World Food Policy dedicated to addressing global food challenges through science and institutional collaboration. This congress is a multidisciplinary initiative that brings together leading scholars from the social sciences—including political science, sociology, economics, and anthropology—agricultural sciences, and nutrition and public health. It will welcome students, non-profit organizations, and policymakers, creating a dynamic space for dialogue and knowledge exchange. It is designed for anyone committed to tackling the complex issues surrounding food security and insecurity from a rigorous, evidence-based perspective. The relevance of our event could not be more critical: armed conflicts are escalating worldwide increasing hunger, climate change continues to disrupt crop production, and the effectiveness of international institutions is increasingly under scrutiny. This congress aims to foster dialogue, share cutting-edge research, and develop actionable strategies to ensure sustainable and equitable food systems for the future.

The primary objective of the 1st International Congress on World Food Policy is to provide comprehensive and up-to-date scientific knowledge about food security and insecurity, examining their effects across diverse temporal and spatial scales. This congress offers an exceptional opportunity to share the growing body of research on these issues, with the participation of national and international experts from multiple disciplines, and to discuss their impact at different levels. The event will convene leading scholars and policymakers to generate actionable insights that can influence both academic research and public policy.

The second objective is to analyze past and current academic literature and policy strategies in response to an expanding range of challenges, addressing issues such as gender perspectives, the right to food, crop modernization, sustainability and practical experiences from the field, among others. Ultimately, it will serve as a dynamic space for knowledge exchange and practical dialogue—benefiting professionals with direct responsibilities, individuals in civil service roles, and other stakeholders committed to making zero hunger a reality.

We look forward to welcoming you on May 8–9, 2026, at University Pablo de Olavide.

Sincerely,

**Alfonso Sánchez Carrasco, PhD**

*President of the Organizing Committee*
*Área de Ciencias Políticas y de la Administración de la Universidad Pablo de Olavide*

# Organizing Committee

## *President*

**Alfonso Sánchez-Carrasco,** Universidad Pablo de Olavide, Área de Ciencias Políticas y de la Administración; Editor-In-Chief, World Food Policy

## *Members*

**Michela Accerenzi,** Fundación ETEA

**Juan José Echanove,** Lead, Right to Food, FAO

**Tony Payan,** Rice University´s Baker Institute & Universidad Autónoma de Ciudad Juárez

**Yolanda Hernández-Albújar,** Universidad de Sevilla

**Miguel Ángel Martín López,** Universidad de Sevilla; Observatorio del Derecho a la Alimentación de España

# Scientific Committee

**Ana Paula Lamoso González,** Universidad Pablo de Olavide

**Sergio Fernández-Artamendi,** Universidad de Sevilla

**Isabel Inguanzo Ortiz,** Universidad de Salamanca

**Manuel Iglesias Cavicchioli,** Universidad Pablo de Olavide

**Beatriz Tomé-Alonso,** Universidad Nacional de Educación a Distancia

**Gloria Martínez-Cousinou,** Universidad de Sevilla

**Ranjan Kumar Guha,** Bangladesh Academy for Rural Development

**Henry G. Hunga,** University of Malawi

**Degefa Tolossa,** Addis Ababa University

**José Manuel Martín,** Fundación ETEA

# Co-Organizers

### *Right to Food Team, FAO*

The Food and Agriculture Organization of the United Nations (FAO) is the specialized agency of the United Nations responsible for leading international efforts to eradicate hunger, improve food security and nutrition, and promote more efficient, inclusive, resilient and sustainable agrifood systems. Within this framework, FAO's Right to Food Team provides technical assistance and policy advice to Member States and other stakeholders to advance the progressive realization of the human right to adequate food. Its work includes strengthening public policies, developing capacities, supporting monitoring and accountability mechanisms, and promoting access to justice and human rights-based approaches in food security and nutrition policies and programs.

### *Policy Studies Organization*

The Policy Studies Organization (PSO) is a non-profit, non-governmental organization dedicated to advancing scholarship and fostering multidisciplinary dialogue on a broad spectrum of policy issues. Through academic journals, books, and conferences, PSO aims to support those involved in the development and evaluation of policy. Originally established as an extension of the American Political Science Association, PSO was created to serve scholars from diverse fields who share an interest in the study and discussion of public and organizational policy.

### *World Food Policy*

World Food Policy (WFP) is a multidisciplinary academic journal published semiannually by Wiley, dedicated to disseminating research focused on food security. The journal places particular emphasis on contemporary issues closely linked to food security, such as climate change, gender equity, armed conflicts, and both national and international policies, among others. WFP is aimed at a broad and diverse audience, including students, scholars, sector professionals, and readers with an interest in the field of food security.

### *Area of Political Science and Public Administration, Universidad Pablo de Olavide*

This year (2026) marks the 20th anniversary of the Political Science and Public Administration program. As part of the celebrations, we are partnering with PSO, WFP, and FAO to host the First International Conference on Food Policy. The event will bring together leading experts from academia, international organizations, NGOs, and policymaking circles, and will feature ten thematic panels covering a range of sociopolitical, health-related, and food security issues.

# Co-organizers and partner organizations

# Keynote Speakers

# Strengthening Food Governance through the Right to Food: Human Rights-Based Approaches for Resilient and Inclusive Agrifood Systems

**Juan Echanove**

*Lead, Right to Food*
*Food and Agriculture Organization of the United Nations (FAO)*

Agrifood systems are at the center of many of today's most pressing global challenges: hunger and malnutrition, climate change, conflict, inequality, unhealthy diets, environmental degradation and loss of trust in public institutions. This intervention argued that the right to adequate food is not merely a legal concept or a moral aspiration, but a practical governance framework for transforming agrifood systems in ways that are more resilient, inclusive and centered on human dignity.

The right to food helps shift the focus from food as a commodity or a question of supply alone towards food as a matter of entitlement, accountability, and public responsibility. It asks whether all people can access adequate, safe, nutritious, culturally acceptable, and sustainable food in dignity, and whether laws, policies, institutions, markets, and budgets are organized around people's needs, especially those most affected by exclusion and food insecurity.

A human rights-based approach strengthens food governance by placing participation, accountability, non-discrimination, transparency, empowerment, human dignity, and rule of law at the center of decision-making. It transforms people from passive beneficiaries into rights holders, and States from voluntary providers into duty bearers. It also helps connect fragmented policy areas (nutrition, land, labor, gender equality, climate resilience, biodiversity, social protection, public procurement, conflict prevention, and access to justice) within a coherent governance framework.

The intervention highlighted that many contemporary food crises are not caused by absolute scarcity, but by systems that produce exclusion, unhealthy food environments, and structural inequality. Hunger and obesity increasingly coexist, often affecting the same vulnerable communities. Children are exposed to aggressive marketing of ultra-processed foods, while healthy diets remain unaffordable for many families. These are not only individual choices, but governance failures requiring public action, regulation, and accountability.

Examples from different countries (e.g., Brazil, Chile, Mexico, India) show how food systems can be changed through deliberate governance choices, including front-of-pack nutrition labelling, regulation of food marketing to children, school feeding programs, public procurement linked to small-scale producers, local food strategies, and food policy councils. These experiences demonstrate that food systems are shaped by law, policy, institutions, resources, and power, and can therefore be redirected towards public interest and human wellbeing.

The right to food is also essential for addressing resilience, gender equality, climate justice, mental health, conflict, and access to justice. Resilient food systems are not only efficient; they are inclusive, accountable, and trusted. Women, Indigenous Peoples, small-scale producers, displaced communities, and marginalized groups must be recognized as central actors in food systems transformation.

Ultimately, strengthening food governance through the right to food means placing people, dignity, and accountability at the center of agrifood systems. It is not only about producing more food, but about building systems that nourish people, protect ecosystems, reduce inequality, enable participation, and secure a more just future.

# The Role of AECID in Promoting Respect, Protection, and Fulfilment of the Human Right to Food

**María Emma Orejudo Prieto de los Mozos**

*Subdirectora de Transición Ecológica, Agua y Lucha contra el Hambre y Oficina del Fondo de Cooperación para Agua y Saneamiento; Dirección de Cooperación Sectorial, Europea y Multilateral; Agencia Española de Cooperación Internacional para el Desarrollo (AECID) Ministerio de Asuntos Exteriores, Unión Europea y Cooperación*

The State of Food Security and Nutrition in the World (SOFI) 2025 report reveals that more than 2.4 billion people experience food insecurity and 3 billion lack access to a healthy diet, underscoring the urgency of global action. In response, Spain is accelerating its commitment to the Sustainable Development Goals (SDGs) by pledging to raise Official Development Assistance to 0.7% of Gross National Income by 2030. Since 2023, Spanish Cooperation has undergone a comprehensive reform through the approval of the Law on Cooperation for Sustainable Development and Global Solidarity and the 2024–2027 Master Plan, both supported by broad political and social consensus. This reform has strengthened the cooperation system by integrating decentralized cooperation, civil society, the private sector, and academia, and by establishing new governance bodies such as the High Council for Sustainable Development Cooperation and the Sectoral Conference. It also includes key institutional advances such as the Statute of Cooperation Personnel, the Statute of AECID, and the creation of the Spanish Fund for Sustainable Development (FEDES), which enhances flexibility and expands financial cooperation. Complementing this framework, the Feminist Strategy (2025) promotes gender equality and the empowerment of women and girls, while the Multilateral Policy Strategy (2026) strengthens global governance, climate action, and food security through a human rights-based approach. The OECD has highlighted Spain's leadership in this context, noting that despite a global decline in ODA, Spain reached a 15-year high of €4.55 billion in 2025. At the international level, the Fourth UN Conference on Financing for Development (2025) produced the Seville Commitment, which promotes sustainable investments in agri-food systems and green fiscal policies.

Within this framework, the Spanish Agency for International Development Cooperation (AECID) places the Human Right to Adequate Food at the core of its action, promoting sustainable production and resilience through agroecology while recognizing that hunger is fundamentally a political issue. AECID supports public policies in partner countries, humanitarian initiatives, and rural development, with a strong emphasis on the role of rural women as key agents of change, advocating for their access to productive resources and land ownership. Spain maintains strategic alliances with major international organizations such as the FAO, WFP, IFAD, and GAFSP, contributing significant funding, and uses FEDES to support initiatives like Kuali and Huruma, which foster financial inclusion and sustainable agrifood value chains. Looking ahead, AECID is coordinating the development of a new Right to Food – Zero Hunger Strategy to guide Spanish cooperation efforts in ensuring access to poor developmental outcomes, and reduced economic mobility.

Addressing food insecurity requires moving beyond isolated interventions toward coordinated, data-driven, and community-centered solutions that recognize the interconnectedness of health, economics, infrastructure, and policy. Sustainable food systems must integrate strategies that promote economic opportunity, transportation access, fair wages, culturally responsive nutrition programs, medically tailored food interventions, and strong community partnerships. Equally important is the meaningful engagement of communities in identifying priorities, shaping interventions, and informing policies that directly affect their well-being. Data-informed decision-making and cross-sector collaboration are critical to developing scalable and sustainable solutions capable of addressing both immediate nutritional needs and the broader structural determinants of food insecurity.

Ultimately, food security must be recognized as a global public health and human rights priority. When food is treated as foundational to life rather than as a privilege or isolated commodity, efforts can shift from merely managing scarcity toward building the conditions necessary for health, resilience, stability, dignity, and opportunity for all communities. Achieving lasting change will require collective global commitment, sustained adequate, healthy, and dignified food for all and advancing toward SDG 2. Finally, AECID strongly condemns the use of hunger as a weapon of war and calls for compliance with UN Security Council Resolution 2417, reaffirming its ethical and legal commitment to protecting the right to food in all contexts.

# Food is Life: A global call to address food insecurity through systems change and community-centered action

**Luz María Garcini, PhD., MPH**

*Rice University*

Food insecurity remains one of the most urgent and complex public health challenges worldwide. Although food is foundational to human survival, health, and well-being, more than 266 million people globally continue to experience uncertain, unstable, or inadequate access to nutritious food. Importantly, food insecurity is not confined to regions experiencing famine or extreme scarcity; it is also prevalent in economically prosperous nations and urban centers where structural inequities, rising costs of living, and limited access to affordable nutritious foods continue to undermine health and quality of life. This presentation, delivered at the World Food Policy Conference at Universidad Pablo de Olavide in Seville, Spain, examined food insecurity as a multidimensional systems issue shaped by social, economic, political, and environmental determinants.

Across global contexts, food insecurity manifests in diverse but interconnected ways. In some communities, it presents through food shortages and malnutrition, while in others it emerges through the overconsumption of low-cost, calorie-dense, nutrient-poor foods driven by economic instability, transportation barriers, inadequate infrastructure, and limited access to healthy food environments. Despite these differing manifestations, common patterns persist worldwide: families forced to choose between affordability and nutrition, communities disproportionately impacted by disinvestment and poverty, and children whose developmental trajectories and future opportunities are shaped by inequitable social conditions.

This work emphasized that food insecurity should not be understood as the consequence of individual behaviors or personal failure, but rather as the product of systemic failures that perpetuate inequities across generations. Fragmented food systems, policy misalignment, inadequate infrastructure, insufficient investment in prevention, unstable economic conditions, and the absence of disaggregated community-level data continue to limit effective responses and widen disparities globally. These structural barriers disproportionately affect marginalized populations and contribute to downstream physical and mental health consequences, including cardiometabolic disease, chronic stress, investment, and systems-level transformation grounded in equity, accountability, and measurable long-term impact.

# Abstracts

## (Oral Presentations)

## Food Policy and Governance I

Discussant: **Dr. Daniel Coq**, *Universidad de Sevilla*

# What do city food networks offer? Resources for sustainable food policy in Brazilian cities

**Feilpe Jardim**

*Tilburg University, Netherlands*

**Giulia Bazzan**

*Tiliburg University, Netherlands*

This study identifies the resources offered by city food networks to Brazilian cities integrating sustainability into their local food policies, motivated by the recognition that global food systems are major drivers of environmental, social, and economic instability while also being increasingly vulnerable to climate change and global crises, positioning cities as central actors in fostering systemic resilience through local, community-driven solutions; by engaging in global, regional, and national networks, cities facilitate knowledge exchange and policy innovation, yet a research gap persists regarding the empirical mapping of city food networks in post-colonial states and comparative evidence on the resources they provide, which this research addresses. The Brazilian case study is based on exploratory qualitative research, including 21 semi-structured interviews with representatives from local, state, and national governments, city food networks, academia, NGOs, and intergovernmental bodies, with thematic analysis focusing on seven major capital cities—Belo Horizonte, Curitiba, Fortaleza, Porto Alegre, Recife, Rio de Janeiro, and São Paulo —representing approximately 27 million inhabitants (around 13% of the national population); these cities participate formally or informally in multiple networks such as the Milan Urban Food Policy Pact, C40, United Nations SDG Cities, United Nations Local2030 Coalition, City Food, Mercociudades, Urban Laboratory for Public Food Policies, and Feeding Cities. Preliminary findings show that city food networks provide five essential types of resources for integrating sustainability into local food policy: human capital (mobilizing political will, expertise, and internal trust), monetary assets (unlocking funding, investments, and trade partnerships), intellectual property (sharing data, toolkits, and policy blueprints), reputational standing (enhancing visibility, prestige, and external trust), and governance (enabling cross-sectoral collaboration through transversal commitments aligning food systems with climate, health, gender, and equity agendas, while positioning cities as actors in urban diplomacy capable of bypassing federal channels to influence global governance); however, networks do not directly provide natural resources (land, water, soil, seeds) or structural resources (buildings, vehicles, equipment, hardware), although these may be indirectly accessed through funding or knowledge. Being part of multiple networks facilitates sustainability integration, yet challenges persist, including weak horizontal integration across municipal departments, absence of dedicated coordinators for knowledge sharing across overlapping networks, and lack of alignment between local governance structures in post-colonial contexts and global network agendas; additional constraints include the absence of standardized impact indicators, language barriers in international engagement, and bureaucratic burdens in cooperation and fundraising processes, all of which limit the transformation of sustainability from a symbolic commitment into a lasting component of local food governance.

# Food Policy in Poland (2020–2025): Intersectoral fragmentation & Milti-level governance challenges

**Leszek Szczepaniak**

*University of Warsaw, Poland*

Food policy has gained increasing relevance as a public policy domain connecting public health, agriculture, climate change, and social welfare; however, Poland has not developed an explicit and coherent national food policy framework. This paper analyzes food policy in Poland between 2020 and 2025, focusing on intersectoral fragmentation and multi-level governance (MLG) challenges that constrain the development of integrated and strategic policymaking. The study is grounded in an MLG perspective and employs qualitative policy and document analysis, drawing on national strategies, legislative acts, governmental programs, and official policy documents addressing food-related issues during this period. The analysis examines how responsibilities related to food systems are distributed across sectors and governance levels, and how this institutional configuration shapes coordination capacity and long-term planning. The findings reveal persistent intersectoral fragmentation, with food-related responsibilities dispersed across policy domains such as agriculture, public health, social policy, and environmental protection, which operate largely in parallel with limited mechanisms for horizontal coordination. As a result, food policy in Poland functions as a collection of sector-specific interventions rather than as an integrated public policy domain, a condition further reinforced by multi-level governance arrangements dividing competencies among the European Union, central government, and subnational authorities. Although food-related issues are addressed at each level, weak vertical coordination limits the emergence of a coherent national policy approach, a problem compounded by the absence of a single strategic document explicitly defining food policy objectives. The analysis also highlights the weak institutionalization of food policy within the political process, where food-related challenges tend to appear as secondary issues within broader sectoral agendas rather than as a distinct, strategically coordinated priority. This limits the capacity to address cross-sectoral challenges such as dietary health inequalities, food system resilience, and long-term sustainability. Overall, the Polish case illustrates how intersectoral fragmentation and multi-level governance complexity hinder the development of integrated food policy, contributing to broader debates by showing how institutional dispersion and limited coordination capacity shape policy outcomes in contexts lacking a formally articulated food policy framework.

# Reducing Leakages in Food-Based Safety Nets: Evidence from India's 'Right to Food' Law

**Raghav Puri**

*Cornell University, United States of America*

**Prabhu Pingali**

*Cornell University, United States of America*

Leakage or diversion of food grains from in-kind food-based safety nets (FBSNs), whether through corruption or operational inefficiencies, is a major hurdle to the effective implementation of these programs. While cash transfers have become a popular way to deliver food benefits, many countries such as India, Indonesia, and Egypt continue to provide in-kind food transfers. Estimating leakages and identifying ways to improve the delivery of in-kind transfers can play a pivotal role in increasing food security for low-income households. This study focuses on India's Public Distribution System (PDS), a national FBSN program that provides 5 kg of free food grains to over 800 million individuals (approximately 10 percent of the global population) every month, procured from farmers at fixed prices and distributed through a nationwide network of PDS shops. Previous research has documented substantial leakages across procurement, transportation, storage, and distribution, with estimates indicating that 41 percent of food grains did not reach beneficiaries in 2011–12. Despite this, there have been no updated leakage estimates since then due to delays in official data collection, even as major reforms have been implemented under India's "right to food" law. This gap in consumption data has limited understanding of the program's current effectiveness, which this study addresses using newly released data from the Household Consumption and Expenditure Survey (HCES). The results show that leakage of PDS food grains declined sharply from over 54 percent in 2004–05 to less than 10 percent in 2023–24. This substantial reduction is attributed to two main factors: the expansion of PDS coverage under the "right to food" law, which reduced exclusion errors and opportunities for rent-seeking, and the adoption of technological innovations such as biometric authentication that improved last-mile delivery. These quantitative findings are further supported by qualitative insights from interviews with PDS beneficiaries and administrators, who highlight improvements in transparency, accountability, and overall functioning of the system over the past decade. Together, the evidence suggests that reforms combining institutional expansion and technology can significantly reduce leakage and enhance the effectiveness of large-scale in-kind food transfer programs.

# From Dietary Tradition to Biological Citizenship: The Algorithmic Governance of Hunger in the Digital Era

**Chrysoula Kapartziani**

*National & Kapodistrian University of Athens, Greece*

**Nikos Symvoulidis**

*National & Kapodistrian University of Athens, Greece*

**Eleni Tsatsaroni**

*National & Kapodistrian University of Athens, Greece*

**Nikolina Tsoukala**

*National & Kapodistrian University of Athens, Greece*

**Stathis Arapostathis**

*National & Kapodistrian University of Athens, Greece*

**Periklis Vardakas**

*University of Thessaly, Greece*

**Dimitra Barkouta**

*National & Kapodistrian University of Athens, Greece*

**Vasiliki Karantzavelou**

*National & Kapodistrian University of Athens, Greece*

This paper argues that Intermittent Fasting (IF) applications are not merely lifestyle tools but sophisticated technologies of "biological citizenship." By converting the subjective sensation of hunger into quantifiable metabolic data, these apps redefine the individual's responsibility toward their own health and reconfigure the relationship between the body, technology, and governance. The study examines how diverse social groups in Greece negotiate this emerging form of digital governance, in which bodily autonomy is increasingly mediated by algorithmic "red flags" and forms of scientific validation. A qualitative research design was employed, combining 30 focus groups and 16 semi-structured interviews (N≈90), organized across seven clusters including shift workers, athletes, religious groups, chronic patients, health professionals, and demographic-specific categories. The research was conducted within the MetaBoost project, part of the Clusters of Research Excellence (CREs) and funded by the European Union – NextGenerationEU through the National Recovery and Resilience Plan "Greece 2.0." Data were analyzed using MAXQDA software through an inductive thematic coding framework to identify patterns related to digital trust, bodily surveillance, and socio-technical expectations. The findings reveal a shift from "voluntary" to "algorithmic" discipline, marked by the emergence of the "biological citizen," particularly among high-risk groups such as diabetics and cancer survivors, who increasingly expect applications to act as "digital bridges" for medical oversight. At the same time, forms of "involuntary fasting" driven by precarious labor conditions are paradoxically reframed by applications as proactive health practices. While some participants embrace the datafication of the body, others highlight risks of "quantification blindness," referring to the inability of algorithms to capture the complexity of human metabolism and the cultural significance of shared eating practices. The study concludes that IF applications enact a co-production of health and technology, in which the right to food security is being reframed as a right to "data-driven wellbeing." In this context, biological citizenship involves a willingness to trade privacy for perceived algorithmic safety, particularly when technologies carry the symbolic legitimacy of academic and clinical validation. These dynamics underscore the need for policy frameworks that address digital food governance, ensuring that such transformations do not deepen health inequalities or undermine the human dimensions of dietary experience.

Discussant: **Dr. Yolanda Hernández-Albújar,** *Universidad de Sevilla*

# Identification of Women's Roles in Food Autonomy Initiatives through Their Participation in Urban and Peri-Urban Agriculture Processes in Different Localities of Bogotá, Colombia

**Ammi Portillo Rueda**

*Universidad de Almería, Spain*

The purpose of this study was to identify the roles of women in food autonomy initiatives through their participation in urban and peri-urban agriculture (UPA) processes across different localities of Bogotá, Colombia. The study is based on the recognition that food autonomy encompasses processes related to food production, access, and consumption, as well as the symbolic and cultural dimensions associated with food systems. In this context, UPA emerges as a strategy that contributes to strengthening food autonomy in response to the inequalities and food-related challenges present within the city.

The research was conducted through a descriptive cross-sectional study employing a mixed-methods approach and a non-probabilistic convenience sampling strategy. The sample consisted of 33 urban and peri-urban women farmers from various localities of Bogotá. Data collection was carried out using surveys, semi-structured interviews, in-depth interviews, and focus group workshops. The information obtained was subsequently analyzed using qualitative data management software, including NVivo. The findings revealed that participants ranged in age from 24 to 66 years and were predominantly characterized by limited economic resources and low-income levels. Furthermore, the most significant roles identified among the women were associated with caregiving activities, particularly those of mother, homemaker, and spouse.

However, participation in urban gardens enabled a reconfiguration of their identities by incorporating roles related to agriculture, community leadership, and food production. The qualitative analysis demonstrated that territory holds an important symbolic dimension for participants, being perceived as a space for personal fulfillment, the construction of community ties, and the strengthening of food-related practices. Likewise, urban gardens were recognized as settings that facilitate the transmission of food traditions and customs, promote food autonomy, and foster the development of social relationships.

In response to the research question, it is concluded that women play fundamental roles as food producers, caregivers, facilitators of social cohesion, and community agents. Their participation in urban and peri-urban agriculture processes contributes to food access and availability, generates positive impacts in the socioeconomic, environmental, and food-related spheres, and strengthens the sustainability of food systems. Nevertheless, inequalities derived from persistent cultural patterns continue to place women in disadvantaged positions, highlighting the need for further analysis from a gender perspective and for greater recognition of their contribution to food autonomy.

# Convergence between Land Tenure Reform and Agricultural Policies: Towards Sustainable Food Sovereignty in Morocco

**Bouchra Fouad**

*Universidad Pablo de Olavide, Spain*

This paper analyzes the critical intersection of land tenure, gender equality, and food security in Morocco, focusing on the case of the mobilization of Soulaliyate women. Gender equality in rural contexts goes beyond the realm of fundamental rights to emerge as a macroeconomic imperative: it is an essential driver of national food security. This premise is strongly supported by empirical evidence from the Food and Agriculture Organization of the United Nations (FAO), whose *State of Food and Agriculture* (2011) report identifies gender inequality as a structural cause of low agricultural productivity in developing countries. Although women constitute the backbone of the rural workforce, their limited access to productive resources and development opportunities systematically constrains farm productivity. Among these barriers, the most critical is their exclusion from legal land ownership, which prevents access to credit, subsidies, technology, and strategic decision-making, thereby undermining the food resilience of the entire nation. This dynamic is exemplified in the case of Soulaliyate women, members of ethnic communities living on collective lands, whose historical exclusion from rights of use and decision-making—codified during the French Protectorate in 1919—represented not only a social injustice but also a structural inefficiency in national agricultural development. With the erosion of traditional patriarchal protection mechanisms, rural women were left in a vulnerable position that limited the productive capacity of their communities. Through the analysis of the mobilization of Soulaliyate women and the implementation of Law 62-17 in 2019, this paper argues that the legal empowerment of women is a necessary condition for food sovereignty. This perspective reframes collective land as a strategic socio-economic asset, whose governance is crucial for national sovereignty in a context of climate crisis and market volatility. By granting women legal security, the transition is enabled from being "courtesy-protected" subjects to fully recognized rights-holders, thereby unlocking access to credit and technical investment and fostering more resilient, diversified, and livelihood-oriented agricultural systems capable of addressing current economic and environmental challenges.

# Experiencing, Exercising, and Resignifying Territory: Contributions of Peasant Women from Antioquia (Colombia) to Food Security Policies

**André Aparecido Medeiros**

*Universidade de São Paulo, Brazil*

**Maria da Penha Costa Vasconcellos**

*Universidade de São Paulo, Brazil*

In Colombian rural territories historically marked by armed conflict, structural marginalization, and the impacts of the COVID-19 pandemic, food insecurity has been determinedly countered through the leadership of peasant women. This study aims to analyze how the daily agroecological practices of women's collectives in Antioquia not only guarantee local subsistence but also serve as innovative tools and bridges for formulating more effective, inclusive, and territorially adapted Food and Nutritional Security and Sovereignty (FNSS) policies.

The research adopted a qualitative and interdisciplinary approach, grounded in phenomenology and humanistic geography. Observational and inquisitive fieldwork was conducted in four locations within the department of Antioquia (San Antonio de Prado, Marinilla, San Cristóbal, and Granada), alongside five associations and corporations of peasant women. Data collection involved participant observation, semi-structured interviews with leaders and members, territorial transects, collective memory circles, and local narrative analysis. Field experiences evidenced that local agroecological practices – such as the implementation of home and community gardens, short marketing circuits (Peasant Markets), and heirloom seed banks – mitigated the immediate food crisis and ensured self-sufficiency. By transcending domestic spaces, these women evolved from "silent producers" into agents of political advocacy. As a practical result of this agency, community-based knowledge generated institutional innovations, such as the project in Granada that enabled public procurement of family farming products for school meals, replacing industrialized goods. Furthermore, the rural movement led by these women influenced the subnational state apparatus, ensuring their field experiences were integrated as strategic pillars in long-term legal instruments, notably the Twelve-Year Food and Nutritional Security Plan (PDSAN 2020-2031) and the Departmental Agroecology Plan of Antioquia (PDEAA 2023-2040).

The experience of the collectives in Antioquia demonstrates that a sustainable response to the agrifood crisis depends on transitioning from top-down, welfare-oriented state approaches to sovereignty models built "from below." Lessons learned on the ground reveal that peasant women are indispensable architects in reconfiguring institutional responses to hunger. Recognizing their local epistemologies and directly integrating their resilience tactics into public policy constitutes the most effective path toward designing food security guidelines that promote gender equity, territorial peace, and true sustainability in rural communities.

Note: This study was financed in part by the Coordenação de Aperfeiçoamento de Pessoal de Nível Superior - Brasil (CAPES) - Finance Code 001.

# Pathways to Wellness: Advancing Food Access and Nutrition among Immigrant Mothers in the United States

**Luz Maria Garcini**

*Rice University, United States of America*

**Tony Payan**

*Rice University/UACJ, United States of America & México*

**Anjelica Martínez**

*Rice University, United States of America*

**Katherine Pérez**

*Rice University, United States of America*

**Diego Maríquez-Robles**

*Rice University, United States of America*

Background: Hunger and food insecurity are widespread and pressing concerns for maternal well-being, with significant implications for maternal health outcomes. Despite global advances in maternal health, the U.S. maternal mortality continues to rise. In the U.S., immigrants comprise a considerable proportion of the population; however, they face high rates of food insecurity and poor nutrition especially those with limited access to services and resources. For many immigrant mothers, these challenges are compounded by histories of trauma, limited access to healthcare, and structural barriers to economic mobility. Identifying prevention and intervention strategies that are culturally and contextually informed is crucial to prevent the detrimental physical and mental health effects of food insecurity and poor nutrition among immigrant mothers and their families. Objective: The proposed project employed mixed methods to conduct an in-depth assessment to understand the food and nutrition needs of immigrant mothers in the U.S., and to identify relevant protective factors to guide prevention and intervention efforts. Methods: In collaboration with an established network of community partners, multi-source data were gathered from June to December 2025 among key informants (n = 25), pregnant and postpartum immigrant mothers (n = 153), and their U.S.-born counterparts (n = 76). In-person interviews facilitated data collection in culturally and contextually informed ways. Mother also provided biomarkers of health and disease risk for close comparison of subjective and objective health. Data gathered included information on sociodemographic profiles, migration history, food access and nutrition, physical and mental health outcomes, non-medical drivers of health, and protective health resources and mechanisms. Results: Hunger and food insecurity disproportionately affect immigrant mothers across pregnancy and postpartum, positioning them as a central determinant of maternal health. Qualitative findings highlighted economic strain, limited family support, inadequate social infrastructure, language misalignment, and limited access to culturally-appropriate nutrition guidance as sociodemographic barriers. Quantitative preliminary results showed that food insecurity was linked to physical health satisfaction ($b = -.09$, $p = .03$), high-risk pregnancy symptoms, ($b = .23$, $p = .01$), high psychological stress ($b = .30$, $p = .01$), reduced quality of life ($b = -.09$, $p = .01$) and increased anxiety symptoms ($b = .23$, $p = .002$). Food insecurity was more prevalent among larger immigrant households: 50% with one or two children reported food insecurity, compared with nearly two-thirds (64%) with three or more children ($p = .03$), and among mothers with job instability and lower incomes ($b = -.003$, $p = .001$). These preliminary findings underscore the urgent need for sustained funding, policy action, and community-based interventions that address hunger and food insecurity as a central pathway to improving immigrant maternal health in the U.S. Conclusions: Immigrant mothers face heightened hunger and food insecurity risk across pregnancy and postpartum, stemming from compounding sociodemographic barriers with severe implications for adverse physical and mental health outcomes. Preliminary findings highlight recommendations for culturally responsive interventions, including sustained cross-sector collaboration responsive to the stage-specific needs; embedding nutrition assistance navigation, education, and support within interventions developed in collaboration with trusted community spaces, using minimally intrusive data infrastructures.

# Women's Empowerment and Reduction of Chronic Malnutrition Through a Gender-Sensitive Multisectoral Approach in Rural Mali

**Eva Iráizoz**

*Action Against Hunger, Spain*

**Caroline Colette André**

*Action Against Hunger, Spain*

**Malika Fedala**

*Action Against Hunger, Spain*

**Mamadou Diepkile**

*Action Against Hunger, Spain*

**Sangaré Mama**

*Action Against Hunger, Spain*

**Mohamadou Diagana**

*Action Against Hunger, Spain*

**Antonio Vargas-Brizuela**

*Action Against Hunger, Spain*

The project "Integrated Fight Against Chronic Malnutrition in Mali" (2021–2026), implemented by Action Against Hunger and local partners in four districts of Mali (Kayes, Kita, Bafoulabé, Sikasso), was based on a central premise—women's autonomy is a key determinant of both food security and maternal and child health; the objective was to improve the nutritional status of girls, adolescents, and women through a multisectoral approach that simultaneously addressed access to essential sexual and reproductive health (SRH) services, care and healthy feeding practices, improvements in WASH infrastructure, and the strengthening of women's decision-making power and economic autonomy, and this capitalization study analyzes how this approach contributed to improving indicators in nutrition and health, food security, WASH, and economic autonomy while mitigating chronic malnutrition and gender inequalities. Materials and Methods: A mixed-methods approach was applied, based on a survey (n = 301), 76 focus groups, and a documentary review of the project since 2021; the analysis followed a theory of change integrating indicators of autonomy (decision-making power, control over income, access to resources), health/SRH, and nutrition/WASH, measuring variations in service coverage, adoption of key practices, and changes in community structures related to gender. Results: The project recorded significant improvements in SRH, with the use of modern family planning methods increasing from 28% to 66%, complete prenatal consultations from 26% to 75%, and facility-based deliveries from 82% to 88%, while decision-making autonomy over personal health rose from 4% to 23%; in nutrition/WASH, separate latrines for girls were achieved in 100% of participating schools, minimum dietary diversity reached 66% among women and 76% among children aged 6–23 months, and exclusive breastfeeding increased to 43%, with areas where women participated more in community committees and intra-household decision-making showing better indicators; in terms of economic autonomy, 84% of women's groups gained secure access to land, agricultural productivity increased with the majority of production used for sale, average female income reached 40,990 FCFA per month, and 69% of women reported mastering basic financial management tools through savings and credit associations, although only 33% participated in decisions over household resources and 50% controlled their own income, reflecting persistent structural barriers such as patriarchal norms, information gaps, and unequal control of resources. Conclusions: The study demonstrated that progress translates into sustainable impacts when accompanied by real increases in women's decision-making power and revealed clear synergies between secure land access, women's economic capacity, service utilization, dietary diversification, and maternal and child health; gender equality is not a complementary outcome but a necessary condition for breaking the intergenerational cycle of chronic malnutrition.

Discussant: **Dr. Sergio Fernández-Artamendi**, *Universidad de Sevilla*

# The Mental Health Toll of Hunger: The Interplay of Trauma, Geography, and Food Insecurity among Latino Immigrants in the U.S. and Mexico

**Luz Maria Garcini**

*Rice University, United States of America*

**Tony Payan**

*Rice University/UACJ, United States of America & México*

**Sabrina Cuauro**

*Rice University, United States of America*

**Cecilia Colunga Rodríguez**

*Rice University, United States of America*

**Mario Angel González**

*Rice University, United States of America*

Food insecurity is a potent toxic stressor with profound implications for public health and migration patterns; while it often acts as a driver of forced migration—defined as the compulsory movement of people due to conflict, violence, or disaster—it is also a frequent consequence of the migration journey and resettlement. For Latino immigrants, food insecurity represents a significant nutritional risk that disrupts dietary patterns, leading to malnutrition and an increased risk of chronic disease, a situation exacerbated in the U.S. by structural barriers such as financial instability, limited transportation, and restricted access to social safety nets; importantly, the prevalence of food insecurity, barriers to food access, and related health impacts vary significantly across geographic and sociopolitical contexts. Objective: This mixed-method study aims to examine how exposure to food insecurity and trauma influences quality of life and psychological distress among Latino immigrants residing in the U.S. and Mexico. Methods: Using purposive sampling, one-on-one semi-structured interviews and biomarker collection were conducted with 348 Latino immigrants across community settings in both countries. Results: The prevalence of food insecurity was markedly higher among participants in Mexico (87%) compared to those in the U.S. (45%); qualitative findings identified key barriers to food access in the U.S., including high costs, limited availability of fresh or organic food, and insufficient time for meal preparation. High rates of trauma were observed across the sample, with 97% of participants in Mexico and 76% in the U.S. reporting at least one lifetime traumatic event. Hierarchical regression analyses showed that for quality of life, the initial model accounted for 42% of the variance, and the inclusion of food insecurity in Step 2 significantly improved the model, explaining an additional 9.0% of variance ($\Delta R^2 = .090$, $p < .001$), with food insecurity emerging as the strongest unique predictor of reduced quality of life ($\beta = -0.38$, $p < .001$); for psychological distress, the initial model explained 52% of the variance, and adding food insecurity increased explanatory power by 5.0% ($\Delta R^2 = .050$, $p < .001$), although trauma remained the primary predictor ($\beta = -0.41$, $p < .001$). Conclusions: These findings demonstrate that food insecurity is a central driver of diminished quality of life beyond trauma exposure, underscoring the mental health burden of inadequate food access; from a policy perspective, this suggests that addressing hunger is not solely a nutritional intervention but a critical strategy for improving mental health and overall well-being, while also highlighting geographic differences in social determinants of health and the need for globally informed, context-sensitive public health interventions and policies.

# Socioeconomic, Health and Dietary Determinants of Food Insecurity in Northern Ghana: A Mixed-effects Models and Machine Learning-based SHAP Analysis

**Luz Anamar Gonzalez de la Risa**

*University of Alcala, Spain*

**Luis Javier Sánchez Martínez**

*Complutense University & Universitat Oberta de Catalunya, Spain*

**Sherifa Yakubu**

*University for Development Studies, Ghana*

**Miguel Ángel García Arias**

*Acción Contra el Hambre, Spain*

**Bless Ayinnogre Adumbire**

*University for Development Studies, Ghana*

**Anthony Paul Apam**

*University for Development Studies, Ghana*

**Abu-Hiban Halid**

*University for Development Studies, Ghana*

**Martin Nyaaba Adokiya**

*University for Development Studies, Ghana*

**Noemi López Ejeda**

*Complutense University, Madrid, Spain*

Global hunger remains at alarming levels, affecting 2.3 billion people worldwide. According to the latest FAO report on the State of Food Security and Nutrition, the African continent is experiencing the most critical situation, with more than one in five people—around 307 million individuals—facing chronic hunger. Recent official data from Ghana show a food insecurity prevalence of approximately 45%, with marked rural–urban disparities and a strong geographic pattern, as food insecurity is especially severe in the northern regions, affecting about 80% of the population. In this context, this study aims to analyze food insecurity levels in peri-urban areas of Tamale city in northern Ghana, measured using the Food Insecurity Experience Scale (FIES), and to identify its main determinants, including socioeconomic, water, sanitation and hygiene (WASH), and dietary factors. To achieve this, two complementary analytical approaches were applied: mixed-effects models, which account for heterogeneity between locations through random effects, and a Random Forest machine learning algorithm selected based on regression performance to capture non-linear relationships and identify the most relevant predictors. Additionally, SHapley Additive exPlanations (SHAP) values were used to provide interpretable insights into the magnitude and direction of each determinant's contribution.

The results show a very high prevalence of food insecurity among the 447 peri-urban households analyzed, reaching 88.14% for any level of food insecurity (FIES > 0) and 42.28% for moderate to severe food insecurity (FIES > 3). The models reveal strong associations between food insecurity and nutritional, health, and socioeconomic factors. The mixed-effects model indicates that water insecurity (HWISE) is positively associated with FIES ($\beta = 0.18$), while the presence of at least one child with wasting ($\beta = 0.10$) and fever as a comorbidity ($\beta = 0.10$) are also linked to higher levels of food insecurity. In contrast, higher monthly income and increased consumption of staple foods and pulses show a protective effect ($\beta = -0.10$ to $-0.16$). These findings are consistent with the Random Forest results, where health, WASH, and dietary variables emerge as the most influential predictors. SHAP analysis further highlights non-linear effects and household-level heterogeneity, improving both global and local interpretability. Overall, peri-urban areas in northern Ghana face a critical food insecurity situation characterized by complex interactions across multiple dimensions, underscoring the need for coordinated interventions by public and private stakeholders. The combined use of interpretable statistical models and machine learning approaches proves particularly valuable for better understanding and addressing food insecurity.

# Dietary Patterns and Common Mental Disorders in the Context of Food Security

**Elaine Santos**

*Universidade de São Paulo, Brazil*

**Lucas Moura**

*Universidade de São Paulo, Brazil*

**Camila Souza**

*Federal University of Rio Grande do Norte (UFRN), Brazil*

**Gustavo Ferreira**

*Universidade de São Paulo, Brazil*

**Angela Trude**

*New York University*

**Dirce Marchioni**

*Universidade de São Paulo, Brazil*

Diet plays a central role in mental health, both of which are strongly influenced by social and economic factors; therefore, socially vulnerable populations may be more exposed to structural barriers that limit access to healthy foods and, as a result, face a higher risk of depression and anxiety. Adherence to healthy dietary patterns thus depends on ensuring food and nutritional security as part of the human right to adequate food. In this context, this study discusses the results of a systematic review that analyzed the relationship between dietary patterns and common mental disorders in adults, interpreting these findings through the FAO conceptual framework of food security, which includes the dimensions of availability, access, utilization, and stability. The review included studies published between 2010 and 2025 in English, Spanish, and Portuguese, covering cohort, case-control, and cross-sectional designs. Article eligibility was assessed using Rayyan Web®, while methodological quality and risk of bias were evaluated with Joanna Briggs Institute tools. Dietary patterns were classified as "Healthy," "Unhealthy," "Mixed," and "Mixed-alcoholic," and Stata 17.0 software was used to generate forest plots. The findings were subsequently analyzed within the FAO framework to better understand their broader implications.

The results suggest a protective effect of healthy dietary patterns against depression, with 18 out of 20 studies on depression and 3 out of 5 on anxiety showing an inverse association. In contrast, associations with unhealthy dietary patterns were less consistent due to high heterogeneity, with approximately half of the studies reporting no significant relationship. Mixed and mixed-alcoholic dietary patterns were also not consistently associated with common mental disorders. Although the review did not directly assess food insecurity, the FAO conceptual framework provides valuable insights for interpreting these findings, highlighting how food and nutrition security may influence mental health through both biological mechanisms—such as nutritional deficiencies—and social and structural mechanisms, including uncertainty about food access, insufficient food intake, and dependence on food assistance. These results emphasize the broader social determinants shaping dietary patterns and mental health outcomes. Ensuring food and nutrition security emerges as a key strategy for protecting against common mental disorders, requiring equitable availability and sustainable access to diverse, high-quality diets, along with attention to utilization and stability. Future research should further explore social and economic inequalities to better understand the uneven distribution of dietary patterns and common mental disorders across populations.

# Accuracy and Precision Assessment of a Mobile Application Compared to the 24-Hour Recall in Estimating Dietary Intake Using a Standardized Meal as Reference

**Alexandro Martagón**

*Tec de Monterrey, México*

**Natalia Soto-Larios**

*Tec de Monterrey, México*

**Adrián Soto**

*Tec de Monterrey, México*

**Carlos A. Aguilar-Salinas**

*Tec de Monterrey, México*

Non-communicable chronic diseases account for 70% of global deaths and are associated with unhealthy lifestyles and diets. In Mexico, more than 37% of adults and up to 40.4% of adolescents are overweight or obese. The 24-hour recall has long been a useful tool for assessing individuals' caloric intake; however, despite its utility, there is still room for improvement due to memory and perception biases from both patients and health professionals. Given current technological advances, the incorporation of mobile applications into standardized procedures for nutritional assessment is highly relevant. This pilot study compared the use of the METAbolique mobile application with the 24-hour recall method to estimate calories and macronutrients (carbohydrates, proteins, and fats), using a standardized meal as a reference.

The sample consisted of 95 adults (median age 26 years; 54% women). After recording the meal in the application and, the following day, through a 24-hour recall, both records were processed using Food Processor software. METAbolique showed minimal mean biases (+4.6 kcal; −4.7 g CHO; +2.4 g PROT; +3.5 g FAT) and lower RMSE values than the 24-hour recall (39 vs. 108 kcal; 6.7 vs. 10.1 g CHO; 4.3 vs. 8.0 g PROT; 1.6 vs. 8.2 g FAT; $p < 0.01$). Its Bland–Altman limits of agreement were narrower (±211 kcal; ±12–19 g). Age, sex, BMI, and waist circumference did not predict absolute error ($\rho \leq 0.13$; $p > 0.20$). The System Usability Scale (SUS) questionnaire yielded a mean score of 85.3, with more than 90% of ratings classified as "good" or "excellent." METAbolique outperforms the 24-hour recall in accuracy, precision, and usability, supporting its validity as a reliable tool for dietary assessment in clinical and research settings.

# To Eat or to Heal: Food Security Profiles and Health Vulnerability in Central America. A Machine Learning Approach Using Gallup World Poll Data

**Luis Javier Sánchez Martínez**

*Complutense University & Universitat Oberta de Catalunya, Spain*

**Miguel Ángel García Arias**

*Acción Contra el Hambre, Spain*

**Francisco Javier Abarca Álvarez**

*Granada University, Spain*

**Hugo Melgar Quiñonez**

*McGill University, Canada*

**Noemí López Ejeda**

*Complutense University, Spain*

Global hunger remains high, affecting 2.3 billion people worldwide, and the FAO monitors its evolution using the Food Insecurity Experience Scale (FIES), a validated global standard. Evidence from multiple studies indicates that food insecurity is strongly associated with structural vulnerability factors such as poverty, low educational attainment, large household size (three or more children), lack of social support, and poor overall wellbeing. In Central America, food insecurity has worsened due to persistent poverty, inflation, and limited access to food. In this context, this study aims to identify household vulnerability profiles and their association with food insecurity using a Machine Learning (ML) approach applied to Gallup World Poll (GWP) data from Guatemala, Honduras, El Salvador, and Nicaragua between 2014 and 2019, including 24,260 individuals. After preprocessing, a variable selection process was conducted using the Variable Selection Using Random Forest (VSURF) algorithm to identify key predictors of FIES. Subsequently, Self-Organizing Maps (SOM) were applied to cluster households into distinct profiles, and logistic mixed-effects models were used to assess the robustness of the identified clusters.

At the national level, Honduras shows the highest levels of food insecurity, with a departmental mean FIES of 4.11 (95% CI: 3.89–4.34), while Guatemala (3.30; 95% CI: 3.14–3.47), El Salvador (3.15; 95% CI: 2.99–3.31), and Nicaragua (3.31; 95% CI: 3.16–3.46) display more homogeneous patterns. Nine key predictors were identified, including variables related to income, health, financial well-being, communication access, and perceived economic stress. Four distinct household clusters emerged, with clear differences in food insecurity levels, socioeconomic conditions, and health outcomes. The most vulnerable group (Cluster 3) exhibits the lowest income (USD 4,253.60), poorest health index (40.08), and highest food insecurity (FIES: 5.47), reaching levels up to 30 times higher than the most secure group. In contrast, Cluster 1 (5,098 households) shows a markedly different profile, with a low FIES score (1.03), highest income (USD 9,491.49), strong communication access (92.75), and the highest financial (60.37) and personal health (85.00) indices. Logistic mixed-effects models demonstrate strong predictive performance (AUC $\approx$ 0.79), confirming cluster robustness. Overall, the findings highlight a strong link between poor health, low income, and food insecurity, suggesting a reinforcing cycle where healthcare costs exacerbate deprivation. They also demonstrate the value of ML approaches in capturing complex, multidimensional interactions and emphasize the importance of integrated data analysis to support evidence-based policymaking and the continuous improvement of social protection strategies.

## The Right to Food

Discussant: **Juan Echanove**, *FAO*

# The Right to Food for All within Planetary Boundaries: A Critical Assessment of Emergent Policy Frameworks for Just and Sustainable Food Systems

**Ana García Juanatey**

*CEI—University of Barcelona, Spain*

**Luca Volpi**

*Societat Orgànica, Spain*

Achieving global food security while remaining within planetary boundaries is a defining governance challenge of the twentyfirst century, requiring policy frameworks and strategies that are compatible with ecological limits. Current scientific consensus shows that food systems are major drivers of ecological overshoot, highlighting the need to shift from productivist approaches toward longterm ecosystem resilience. However, traditional frameworks such as food security were developed in a context shaped by perceived abundance and the productivist paradigm of the Green Revolution, centered on synthetic fertilizers and yield maximization. Likewise, human rights–based approaches, including the right to food, tend to prioritize present-day obligations and often overlook long-term ecological integrity and intergenerational fairness. Against this backdrop, this article examines two emerging frameworks—intergenerational justice and the bioeconomy—to evaluate their potential contribution to a coherent agenda for realizing the right to food within planetary boundaries.

The study conducts a comparative analysis of international normative frameworks on intergenerational equity and bioeconomy policies and their implications for the right to food. On the one hand, it analyzes key instruments related to intergenerational justice, including the 2023 Maastricht Principles on the Human Rights of

Future Generations and the 2024 United Nations Pact for the Future. On the other hand, it examines the EU Bioeconomy Strategy through the analytical lens of ecological economics and core human rights principles such as accountability and participation. The results reveal a fundamental tension between these frameworks. Intergenerational equity opens pathways for a transformative interpretation of the right to food by integrating foresight and longterm planning into food policies. In contrast, bioeconomy-based frameworks, while offering tools for decarbonization, tend to prioritize growth and efficiency, which may intensify pressures on ecosystems and contribute to breaching planetary boundaries, including biodiversity loss, freshwater depletion, and land-use change. Moreover, their technocratic and top-down orientation raises concerns about their capacity to address the needs of vulnerable populations and to positively support the realization of the right to food.

The findings indicate that achieving the right to food within planetary boundaries requires embedding ecological limits and intergenerational equity into food governance. Intergenerational justice provides critical normative guidance by emphasizing long-term stewardship and the rights of future generations, whereas the bioeconomy—when driven primarily by growth imperatives—risks exacerbating ecological degradation and social inequities. The study argues that bioeconomy strategies must be subordinated to principles of sufficiency and thermodynamic constraints to ensure sustainability. It concludes by proposing an integrated governance model that incorporates tools such as intergenerational impact assessments, ensuring that the development of a biobased economy strengthens rather than undermines the ecological foundations necessary for the realization of the right to food.

# Structural Judicial Protection of the Right to Food in Colombia: The Case of the Wayuu Children in La Guajira

**Diana Guarnizo Peralta**

*Justice and Society DEJUSTICIA, Colombia*

**Julián Gutiérrez-Martínez**

*Justice and Society DEJUSTICIA, Colombia*

**Adriana Carolina Torres Bastidas**

*Justice and Society DEJUSTICIA, Colombia*

Although the right to food is widely recognized in international treaties, legal recognition of this right in courts is still developing. Several tribunals, particularly in the Global South (e.g., Latin America, India, and South Africa), have enforced this right through landmark decisions, thereby increasing consensus on its justiciability. Nevertheless, many questions remain about the impact of judicial decisions on the full realization of the right to food. In Colombia, for instance, the Constitutional Court issued Ruling T-302 of 2017, which addressed the right to food for Wayuu indigenous children in La Guajira on a structural level. The ruling advances the guarantee of this right by ordering the government to ensure minimum fulfillment levels through dialogical remedies. However, nine years after its enactment, the right has not been fully realized. Compliance with structural decisions is generally challenging in most jurisdictions, particularly in countries with weak institutions. What, then, does the experience of Colombia's Constitutional Court with this ruling reveal about the capacity of structural judicial decisions to advance the realization and enforceability of the right to food in the Global South?

Rather than engaging in a comparative analysis, this paper advances a case study with the objective of analyzing the potential impacts of this decision, specifically on the realization of the right to food. It aims to discuss whether this ruling, understood as an example of structural litigation concerning the right to food, has contributed to guaranteeing said right or to advancing on its recognition and enforceability.

Our analysis relies on qualitative data reported in documents produced by state offices, NGOs, and civil society organizations and published within the last nine years. We also consider data from four field visits conducted between 2017 and 2024. Using an autoethnographic approach, we assess the information as researchers of Dejusticia, a Colombian organization that has participated in the litigation and follow-up of the case since its origins in 2017. Finally, we analyze the effects using the matrix proposed by Rodríguez-Garavito and Rodríguez-Franco (2015, 2022), which categorizes effects as direct or indirect and material or symbolic. This results in four categories: direct/material, indirect/material, direct/symbolic, and indirect/symbolic.

Preliminary analysis of the data shows that, besides the low level of compliance regarding direct and indirect material effects—mainly due to the lack of political will and institutional capacity to develop a comprehensive policy to address malnutrition—the decision has been beneficial in the other three categories. These include an increased coalition of activists and organizations influencing the implementation of the decision (indirect and material), recognizing the problem as a human rights issue (symbolic and direct), and the general acknowledgment of the severity of the issue by the public (symbolic and indirect).

By offering an in-depth examination of a landmark case from the Global South that directly addresses the right to food, this study contributes to ongoing scholarly debates on the impacts of structural judicial decisions and engages with existing literature on the judicial enforcement of the right to food.

# Income Dynamics, Food Consumption and the Right to Food among Vulnerable Farming Families in Brazil: A Quantile Regression Analysis

**Lucas Moura**

*University of São Paulo, Brazil*

**Flávia Mori Sarti**

*University of São Paulo, Brazil*

**Carolina Xavier**

*Federal University of São João del-Rei, Brazil*

**Dirce Marchioni**

*University of São Paulo, Brazil*

Understanding the role of income on household food expenditures is fundamental for ensuring the effective realization of the right to adequate food, especially among vulnerable populations in developing countries marked by high inequalities. This study analyses the association between household income and the proportion of food expenditures among vulnerable farming families in Brazil, applying quantile regression models for the period from 2012 to 2023 to capture the distributional heterogeneity and temporal dynamics relevant to food and nutritional security.

The study was based on repeated cross-sectional microdata from 2012 to 2023, at the household level, referring to families whose reference person is an agricultural worker and who are registered in the Unified Registry for Social Programmes (CadÚnico)—the Brazilian national registry of socially vulnerable families—we estimate quantile regression models at $\tau = 0.25$, 0.50, and 0.75, in which the dependent variable is the proportion of household income allocated to food expenditure. This approach allows us to analyze the conditional distribution of the share of the budget allocated to food and capture the heterogeneity in the relationship between income and food expenditure at different points in the distribution. Household income is measured as the average monthly household income, and the models are estimated separately for each year to track temporal changes associated with economic cycles and macroeconomic shocks. All variables were deflated using Brazil's official consumer price index (IPCA).

Across years and quantiles, the income coefficient is negative and highly statistically significant in relation to food expenditures, following Engel's Law. In 2012, estimated elasticities were approximately -0.17 ($\tau = 0.25$), -0.25 ($\tau = 0.50$), and -0.40 ($\tau = 0.75$), indicating a strong decline in the food expenditure share as income increases. By 2014, these magnitudes fell to -0.12, -0.19, and -0.28, respectively, suggesting increased flexibility in consumption and reduced budgetary pressure for food acquisition. During the 2015–2016 economic downturn, elasticities further weakened (e.g., -0.10 at $\tau = 0.25$ and -0.26 at $\tau = 0.75$ in 2016), reflecting constrained adjustment capacity under deteriorating economic conditions. From 2017 to 2019, elasticities stagnated around -0.09 ($\tau = 0.25$), -0.18 ($\tau = 0.50$), and -0.25 ($\tau = 0.75$), indicating entrenched consumption patterns. The 2020–2021 period - the same as the Covid-19 pandemic - led to renewed increases in magnitude, particularly at higher quantiles (e.g., -0.27 at $\tau = 0.75$ in 2020), before partial attenuation to -0.07 at the lower quantile by 2023.

The findings show that income remains a distributionally heterogeneous determinant of food expenditure shares, particularly among vulnerable farming households, with direct implications for the realization of the right to food. Higher elasticities at upper quantiles indicate greater sensitivity to income fluctuations among households under tighter food budget constraints, increasing vulnerability to food and nutritional insecurity during economic and political shocks. Temporal patterns further reveal that macroeconomic instability and institutional crises undermine these households' capacity to secure adequate food, underscoring income support and social protection policies as state obligations to safeguard the right to food.

# Municipalizing the Right to Food: The Role of Municipalities in Implementing International Human Rights Commitments

**Maria Luisa Cannas**

*Donà Viscardini Law Firm, Italy*

The right to food can be considered a paradigmatic example of a "de-centered" human right: its effective realization depends not only on States, but also on a plurality of actors operating at different levels of governance. In particular, although firmly established within international human rights law, the implementation of the right to food remains uneven. Persistent food insecurity and the inability of millions of people to access healthy diets reveal a significant gap between the formal recognition of this right and its concrete realization.

One of the reasons why this gap is still a burden to the effective realization of the right to food can be found in the distance between decision-making processes at an international and national level and the everyday experiences of individuals, a distance that results in policies that are insufficiently adapted to the needs of communities. The situation can be addressed as an "implementation gap" where national legal recognition does not necessarily mean effective local realization.

Stating from this consideration, the presentation examined the emerging role of municipalities in addressing this implementation gap. Due to their proximity to citizens and their direct involvement in social services, urban planning and local policies, municipalities are uniquely positioned to translate international human rights commitments into context-specific actions. In this perspective, local authorities can act as intermediary actors between the legal recognition of the right to food and its enjoyment within communities.

The presentation explored this dynamic through the case study of the City of Bologna, which in 2023 introduced the *ius cibi* (right to food) within the "Metropolitan Food Policy framework" and, subsequently, in 2025 formally integrated the *ius cibi* within its Municipal Statute. This initiative represents one of the first attempts in Italy to formally recognize the right to food at municipal level and to integrate it into local governance strategies. The analysis investigates both the legal significance and the practical implications of this development. The Bologna experience is interpreted as a process of legal localization; whereby international human rights principles acquire practical meaning through local policies. At the same time, the presentation assessed the limits of municipal action: while municipalities can contribute significantly to the realization of the right to food, they cannot replace the primary obligations of States and remain dependent on broader legal, institutional and financial frameworks.

The Bologna experience suggests that the right to food may increasingly operate through a hybrid enforcement model, where implementation depends not only on legal recognition and judicial remedies, but also on governance mechanisms, institutional coordination and local participation. In this regard, the Bologna case also highlights the growing relevance of the concept of "food citizenship" and the role of local communities in shaping food governance.

Finally, the presentation suggested that contemporary debates on the right to food should also reflect on the evolving meaning of "adequate food." In contexts where food insecurity coexists with food waste and unsustainable consumption patterns, the implementation of the right to food may increasingly require attention not only to access and sufficiency, but also to sustainability and responsible food governance; in this context, the mentioned "food citizenship" acquires even more importance.

Discussant: **Dr. Sergio Fernández-Artamendi**, *Universidad de Sevilla*

# Evaluation of the DPP-IV Inhibitory Activity of Novel Peptides from Hemp as an Alternative Therapy for Alzheimer's Disease

**José Antonio Camacho-Muriel**

*Instituto de la Grasa (CSIC), Spain*

**Lucía Jiménez-Alonso**

*Instituto de la Grasa (CSIC), Spain*

**Gabriel García Jiménez**

*Instituto de la Grasa (CSIC), Spain*

**Álvaro Villanueva-Lazo**

*Instituto de la Grasa (CSIC), Spain*

**Lourdes M Varela**

*Instituto de la Grasa (CSIC), Spain*

**Mª del Carmen Millán-Linares**

*Instituto de la Grasa (CSIC), Spain*

Alzheimer's disease is a neurodegenerative disorder characterized by pronounced cognitive impairment, recent memory loss, and progressive deterioration of language and executive functions, largely driven by pathological mechanisms such as β-amyloid plaque accumulation and neurofibrillary tangles in the brain. Recent research highlights a correlation between Alzheimer's disease and type 2 diabetes mellitus (T2DM), as insulin resistance disrupts glucose metabolism and neurotransmitter regulation, promoting inflammation and oxidative stress in neuronal cells. In response, antidiabetic therapies targeting intestinal hormones, particularly dipeptidyl peptidase-IV (DPP-IV) inhibitors, have gained attention due to their ability to increase glucagon-like peptide-1 (GLP-1) levels, enhance insulin secretion, and potentially improve cognitive performance. However, to reduce adverse effects associated with synthetic drugs, research has increasingly focused on natural bioactive compounds. Hemp seed protein hydrolysates, rich in peptides and amino acids, have demonstrated antioxidant, antihypertensive, hypoglycemic, and immunomodulatory properties, making them promising candidates for neuroprotective and antidiabetic applications. Therefore, this study aimed to identify the hemp seed protein hydrolysate with the greatest in vitro DPP-IV inhibitory activity in a cell-free system, and thus the highest potential to enhance insulin secretion and support cognitive function.

Four hemp protein hydrolysates were produced by enzymatic hydrolysis using Bioprotease LA660 under controlled conditions (15, 30, 45, and 60 minutes), and their DPP-IV inhibitory activity was quantified by measuring the release of the fluorophore 7-amino-4-methylcoumarin (AMC) from the substrate H-Gly-Pro-AMC. Enzyme inhibition percentages were used to calculate $IC_{50}$ values, defined as the concentration required to inhibit 50% of DPP-IV activity. Among the hydrolysates, HBIO30 showed the lowest $IC_{50}$ ($0.0059 \pm 0.0012$ mg/ml), followed by HBIO60 ($0.0065 \pm 0.0012$ mg/ml), indicating higher inhibitory potency, while HBIO45 ($0.0088 \pm 0.0025$ mg/ml) and HBIO15 ($0.0092 \pm 0.0082$ mg/ml) required higher concentrations to achieve similar inhibition. Compared to pharmacological GLP-1/DPP-IV inhibitors, which generally require higher concentrations, these lower $IC_{50}$ values suggest a stronger inhibitory capacity of hemp-derived peptides. These findings highlight their potential as effective and safer alternatives to conventional DPP-IV-targeting drugs. In conclusion, hemp seed protein hydrolysates with potent antidiabetic activity were successfully identified, and their strong inhibitory capacity supports their potential as natural and sustainable therapeutic agents for both Alzheimer's disease and type 2 diabetes.

# Autistic and Alexithymic Traits: Impact on Eating Behavior

**Carla María Pérez-Jaén**

*Universidad Loyola Andalucía, Spain*

**Cristian Manuel Olarte-Sánchez**

*Universidad Loyola Andalucía, Spain*

**Emilio Pericet-Caro**

*Universidad Loyola Andalucía, Spain*

**Julieta Sánchez-Bizama**

*Universidad Loyola Andalucía, Spain*

Autism Spectrum Disorder (ASD) is a neurodevelopmental condition characterized by social and communication difficulties, as well as restrictive and repetitive behaviors and interests (American Psychiatric Association [APA], 2022). According to the World Health Organization, approximately 1 in 100 people are autistic (World Health Organization, 2023), and prevalence has increased in recent decades (Flujas-Contreras et al., 2023). Alexithymia, on the other hand, is a personality trait involving difficulties in identifying and understanding emotions (Poquérusse et al., 2018), and it is estimated that about half of autistic individuals also present alexithymia (Kinnaird et al., 2018). Both autism and alexithymia have been linked to eating disorders (EDs), which are characterized by disruptive eating behaviors that negatively affect relationships with food, as well as psychological, social, and physical health (APA, 2022). The prevalence of EDs has also increased (Cano et al., 2022), and studies indicate a high proportion of autistic individuals among those with EDs (Law, 2023), with some suggesting that alexithymia may act as a mediating factor (Adams et al., 2024). Understanding differences in eating behavior across populations is therefore essential to design appropriate interventions, particularly for groups at higher risk of developing EDs. In this context, the present study aims to explore the relationship between autistic traits, alexithymic traits, and eating patterns.

A total of 371 participants completed an online questionnaire including the Dutch Eating Behaviour Questionnaire (DEBQ), the Autism Quotient-10 (AQ-10), and the Toronto Alexithymia Scale (TAS-20). The DEBQ assesses emotional, external, and restrictive eating behaviors; the AQ-10 screens for autistic traits; and the TAS-20 evaluates alexithymia. Pearson correlation analyses were conducted to examine associations between these variables. Results showed a significant positive correlation between autistic traits and emotional eating ($r = 0.155$, $p < 0.003$), but no significant relationship with restrictive eating ($r = 0.051$, $p > 0.05$) or external eating ($r = 0.053$, $p < 0.05$). In contrast, alexithymia was significantly correlated with all three eating patterns: emotional eating ($r = 0.270$, $p < 0.001$), restrictive eating ($r = 0.178$, $p < 0.001$), and external eating ($r = 0.174$, $p < 0.001$). These findings suggest that both autistic and alexithymic traits influence eating behavior, with autistic individuals more likely to exhibit emotional eating, while alexithymia is associated with all types of eating patterns. This may help explain the high prevalence of autism and alexithymia among individuals with EDs and highlights the importance of tailoring interventions to account for the specific needs of neurodivergent populations, rather than relying solely on approaches designed for neurotypical individuals.

# Food Addiction in Late Adolescence: Impact on Social Functioning, Anxiety, and Severe Depression

**Emilio Pericet-Caro**

*Universidad Loyola Andalucía, Spain*

**Cristian Manuel Olarte-Sánchez**

*Universidad Loyola Andalucía, Spain*

**Julieta Sánchez-Bizama**

*Universidad Loyola Andalucía, Spain*

**Carla María Pérez-Jaén**

*Universidad Loyola Andalucía, Spain*

Food addiction (FA) has become an increasingly recognized phenomenon, particularly in individuals struggling with overweight and obesity, characterized by compulsive eating behaviors. Despite the significant effects of interventions targeting dietary changes and physical activity, their long-term success often diminishes. This has led to a growing interest in the psychological mechanisms involved, including the addictive properties of certain foods (Morales & Berridge, 2020; Baik, 2021) and the emotional regulation function of eating (Van Strien, 2018). FA, which is viewed as both a behavioral and substance-related addiction (Meule, von Rezori, & Blechert, 2014), describes a chronic pattern where individuals uncontrollably seek and consume particular foods despite adverse health consequences (Agüera et al., 2015). Evidence of biological (Kupra et al., 2024), psychological, and behavioral similarities between FA and traditional addictions suggests that exploring eating behaviors, such as FA, is critical to understanding obesity's root causes.

This study involved 522 late-adolescent participants (mean age = 19.68). We used the Yale Food Addiction Scale 2.0 (YFAS 2.0) (Gearhardt et al., 2016), adapted to measure food-related addiction symptoms, and the General Health Questionnaire-28 (GHQ-28) (Lobo, Pérez-Echeverría, & Artal, 1986), which assesses anxiety, depression, insomnia, somatic symptoms, and social dysfunction. Adolescents diagnosed with food addiction reported significantly higher levels of anxiety ($p < 0.001$), social dysfunction ($p < 0.001$), and severe depression ($p < 0.001$) compared to their non-addicted peers.

**Food addiction** (FA) is gaining significant attention for its mental and social implications, particularly in adolescents. This study contributes to understanding the broader effects of FA by highlighting its connection to mental health dimensions like anxiety and depression. Further research is needed to validate FA as a clinical condition and develop therapeutic interventions that address its multifaceted nature, incorporating psychological and behavioral strategies. Existing multicomponent interventions, which improve adolescent well-being by promoting healthier habits and involving families and schools, have shown promise (Diao et al., 2020), suggesting that such approaches could serve as a foundation for future therapeutic frameworks.

# Integrated Approaches to Social Protection and Strengthening Food Agency in Contexts of Socioeconomic Exclusion: Evidence from the Solidarity Cards Program

**Beatriz Tamayo-Borrajo**

*Action Against Hunger, Spain*

**Noemí López-Ejeda**

*Action Against Hunger, Spain*

**Sara Tulipani**

*Action Against Hunger, Spain*

**Rafael Tomás-Cardoso**

*Complutense University, Spain*

**Cristina Cozar**

*Action Against Hunger, Spain*

**Lorena Hernández**

*Action Against Hunger, Spain*

**Antonio Vargas-Brizuela**

*Action Against Hunger, Spain*

The relationship between unemployment and the loss of health and well-being is complex and bidirectional and is mediated by food insecurity. In Spain, Action Against Hunger implements the "Solidarity Cards" (SC) program, integrated into its "Vives-Emplea Saludable" (VES) socio-labor insertion pathways, which combines cash transfers with awareness-raising adapted to low-income contexts. The objective of the study was to analyze the effect of these interventions on improving employability, food security, habits, and health among people experiencing socio-economic exclusion.

Within Action Against Hunger's research line "Social innovation in labor market integration: promotion of healthy lifestyles and their impact on employment," a non-controlled/non-randomized community trial was conducted with unemployed adults participating in VES programs across five municipalities in the Madrid region (n = 307), including recipients of the SC program (n = 165) selected based on high vulnerability criteria (e.g., survivors of violence, single-parent families, households with unemployed adults and children, certification of social exclusion). In addition to financial support (€346/month for two months), participants attended tailored food education sessions designed to address individual determinants of poor diets among low-income populations (economic, cognitive-behavioral, psychosocial, and agency-related barriers), in line with Action Against Hunger's technical framework. Indicators of food insecurity (FIES), dietary diversity (HDDS), employability, habits, and self-reported health (Likert scale) were measured at baseline, at program completion, and at least four months after its end.

At baseline, food insecurity affected 52.7% of participants (17.8% moderate/severe) and was associated with low dietary diversity (42.5%) and worse self-reported health and nutrition conditions ($p < 0.001$). After program participation, 28.3% of cases showed significant improvements in food security, and 11.5% exited food insecurity. In the overall group, significant improvements were observed in dietary diversity (vegetables +15.0%, fruits +13.2%, pulses +13.7%), general health (+11.5%), mood (+30.2%), and lifestyle habits (diet +21.3%, physical activity +15.2%, sleep quality +18.9%). In the SC group, significant increases were recorded in the consumption of fresh protein-rich foods (meat +15.7%, fish +23.5%, dairy +13.7%), and up to 80% reported improvements in label reading, reduction of sugars/ultra-processed foods, hydration, and meal planning. Socio-labor insertion rates reached 69.8% in the overall group (56.5% employment) and 52.0% in the SC group (36.8% employment), reflecting greater barriers among highly vulnerable profiles

This integrated model—combining employability pathways, cash transfers, and food education—aligns with a biopsychosocial understanding of health, improves key dimensions of food security alongside dietary diversity, healthy habits, and well-being, and offers a concrete pathway to break the cycle of exclusion–food insecurity–distress, with important programmatic and public policy implications. However, SC recipients continue to face barriers to accessing quality employment, suggesting the need for differentiated support strategies with greater intensity and/or duration.

# Inhibition of Amyloidβ Fibrillation by Hemp Seed Protein Hydrolysates: Influence of Hydrolysis Degree and Peptide Size


**Lucía Jiménez-Alonso**

*Instituto de la Grasa (CSIC), Spain*

**José Antonio Camacho-Muriel**

*Instituto de la Grasa (CSIC), Spain*

**Gabriel García-Jiménez**

*Instituto de la Grasa (CSIC), Spain*

**Álvaro Villanueva-Lazo**

*Instituto de la Grasa (CSIC), Spain*

**Mª del Carmen Millán-Linares**

*Instituto de la Grasa (CSIC), Spain*

**Lourdes M Varela**

*Instituto de la Grasa (CSIC), Spain*


Alzheimer's disease (AD) is a progressive neurodegenerative disorder and one of the leading causes of dementia worldwide. Its pathological hallmarks include extracellular deposition of amyloidβ (Aβ) plaques, intracellular neurofibrillary tangles composed of hyperphosphorylated tau, and sustained neuroinflammation. Among these, the aggregation of Aβ into fibrillar and oligomeric forms is considered a central driver of neuronal toxicity, vascular impairment, and cognitive decline. As there is currently no effective pharmacological cure for AD, interest has grown in preventive and nutritional strategies capable of modulating early pathogenic events.

Plantderived protein hydrolysates have emerged as promising candidates due to their bioactive peptides with antioxidant, antiinflammatory and antiaggregating properties. Hemp seed protein hydrolysates (HPH) in particular stand out because of their favorable amino acid profile, sustainable production, and demonstrated biological activity. This study investigates the capacity of HPH to inhibit Aβ fibril formation and evaluates how hydrolysis duration and peptide size influence this effect.

HPH were produced through enzymatic hydrolysis using Bioprotease LA660 (0.3 AU/g protein) for four controlled durations: 15, 30, 45 and 60 minutes, generating samples HPHBIO15, HPHBIO30, HPHBIO45 and HPHBIO60. Each hydrolysate was subsequently fractionated into highmolecularweight (HMW) and lowmolecularweight (LMW) peptide fractions to assess sizedependent bioactivity. Antiaggregating activity was quantified using the ThioflavinT (ThT) fluorescence assay. Hydrolysates (100 μg/mL), each fraction, and synthetic Aβ (50 μM) were coincubated in the presence of ThT (5 μM) at 37 °C for 96 hours. Fluorescence readings (excitation 420 nm, emission 515 nm) were collected every 24 hours to determine the kinetics of Aβ fibrillation and the inhibitory effects of each treatment. Aβ samples without hydrolysates displayed maximal fibril formation at 48 hours, establishing this time point as the reference for comparison. Among the unfractionated hydrolysates, only HPHBIO15 and HPHBIO30 significantly inhibited Aβ aggregation, reducing fluorescence intensity by 27% and 32% respectively. Fractionated samples revealed a consistent trend: all LMW fractions exhibited inhibitory activity, though with variable magnitude. LMW15 showed the strongest effect (43% reduction), followed by LMW45 and LMW60 (both 33%), while LMW30 showed moderate inhibition (17%). In contrast, HMW fractions displayed minimal or no inhibitory activity, suggesting that smaller peptides are primarily responsible for the antiaggregating effect.

The data indicate that both the degree of hydrolysis and the molecular weight distribution of HPHs significantly modulate their ability to inhibit Aβ fibrillation. Shorter hydrolysis times and lowermolecularweight peptides consistently demonstrated the highest antiaggregating activity. These findings support the potential of hempderived peptides as natural bioactive compounds for earlystage intervention or prevention strategies related to AD pathology, warranting further investigation into their mechanisms and invivo efficacy.

# The Evolution of AI in Research

**Jonathan Ingram**

*Wiley*

*Editor in Chief at Food and Energy Security, John Wiley & Sons Ltd.*

Based on a global survey of over 2,400 researchers, the ExplanAItions 2025 report shows that AI use in research has surged in just one year. Adoption is widespread, but depth of impact is constrained by limited access to specialist tools, growing concerns about accuracy, ethics, and data security, and a lack of institutional guidance. Researchers report clear efficiency gains yet are recalibrating expectations of AI's capabilities. The findings highlight a critical opportunity for publishers and institutions to provide trusted tools, training, and transparent frameworks to enable responsible, transformative AI use in research. This seminar will cover the main findings of the ExplanAItions 2025 report, practical, shared experience with AI as an Editor in Chief, as well as the dos and don'ts of AI use for authors, editor and reviewers. A Q&A will allow space to explore experiences further, including the overall publishing process and tips for success.

## From Field Experiences to Policy I

Discussant: **Dr. Michela Accerenzi**, *Fundación ETEA/Universidad Loyola Andalucía*

# Rethinking School Feeding Beyond the Cafeteria: Lessons and Challenges from the Sustainable Schools Approach in Colombia

**Laura Catherine Arévalo Rivera**

*FAO, Colombia*

School feeding has traditionally been addressed as a food provision program aimed at improving school attendance and retention; however, this approach is insufficient to comprehensively transform the conditions that shape the eating practices of children and adolescents. This paper proposes rethinking school feeding beyond the cafeteria, placing it within the framework of school food environments, understood as the set of political, social, cultural, environmental, and economic factors that influence food-related decisions within educational settings.

The analysis is based on a participatory process of adaptation and piloting of the Sustainable Schools Methodology in Colombia. The findings show that school feeding should be understood as a complex system in which coherence between food provision, educational processes, and regulatory frameworks is decisive. In particular, the role of school shops—as part of the food environment—is highlighted as a key yet still insufficiently addressed space in shaping dietary practices.

The experience demonstrates that participatory approaches support the development of context-specific solutions, strengthen local governance, and contribute to the design of more comprehensive, coherent, and sustainable public policies. Consequently, advancing the realization of the Right to Adequate Food and the Right to Education requires a shift from an assistance-based approach toward policies aimed at the structural transformation of school food environments.

# The Constitutional Debate in Colombia on Protection Areas for Food Production: Analysis of the Relationship between Land Use Planning Public Policy and the Human Right to Food

**Laura Sofía Ramírez Rivero**

*CEPC, Spain*

This article analyzes the constitutional debate in Colombia surrounding protection areas for food production and their relationship with the human right to food as a land-use planning public policy. The study examines the importance of protecting rural land to ensure food security and the sustainability of the country's agri-food systems.

A legal analysis is developed based on national and international normative, doctrinal, and jurisprudential sources related to the right to food and the protection of rural land as land-use planning policies. The study also highlights the territorial effects of the APPA (Areas for the Protection of Food Production) in regions with the highest levels of food insecurity in the country. In addition, it reviews comparative experiences from other states that have implemented mechanisms to protect land designated for food production. Based on this analysis, key elements are identified to understand the connection between the social and ecological function of land, territorial planning, and state obligations regarding the right to food.

Finally, legal arguments are presented in relation to the constitutional proportionality test, as well as the constitutional legitimacy of the policy establishing protection areas for food production—particularly in light of Article 65 of the Political Constitution of Colombia—and its consistency with the State's international obligations to respect, protect, and fulfill the human right to food.

# Intersectoral Governance and Chronic Child Malnutrition: Lessons from Territorial Coordination in Ecuador


**María Pilar Villena-Esponera**

*Universidad internacional de La Rioja, Spain*

**Marta Caballero**

*Universidad internacional de La Rioja, Spain*

**Verónica Condor Bermeo**

*Universidad internacional de La Rioja, Spain*

**María del Mar Rodriguez-Brioso**

*Universidad internacional de La Rioja, Spain*


Chronic child malnutrition (CCM) is one of the main challenges facing food systems and public health in certain countries, requiring intersectoral responses that integrate interventions in health, social protection, education, the environment, among others. In Ecuador, Cantonal Intersectoral Roundtables (MICs) have been established as local coordination spaces where different sectors work together to promote actions aimed at preventing chronic child malnutrition [1]. However, the effectiveness of these spaces depends on institutional capacities, contextual opportunities, and the motivation of the actors involved. The objective of this study was to analyze, from the perspective of MIC participants, the facilitators and barriers influencing intersectoral cooperation, in order to generate evidence-based recommendations to strengthen the implementation of multi-level public policies.

A qualitative study with a comprehensive-interpretative approach was conducted, based on six focus groups involving 18 participants from operational MICs in different regions of Ecuador. The sample included representatives from national ministries, decentralized autonomous governments, and community actors. A non-probabilistic purposive sampling strategy was used, prioritizing experience in intersectoral coordination processes and territorial diversity. Data were analyzed using thematic analysis, organizing findings according to the COM-B model (Capability, Opportunity, and Motivation) [2], linked to behaviors that influence intersectoral cooperation in the prevention of child malnutrition. Participation in the study was strictly voluntary and informed, and the protocol was reviewed and approved by the Ethics Committee of the Universidad Internacional de La Rioja (Ref. PI: 033_2025).

The study highlights the potential of MICs as formal coordination spaces that facilitate resource sharing, alignment of priorities, and the adaptation of national policies to local contexts. Collaboration with community actors, universities, and non-governmental organizations strengthens social legitimacy and the effectiveness of interventions. Motivation among participants is reinforced by tangible results, such as improved access to services and positive impacts on families, as well as through continuous training and the ethical commitment of staff. However, the findings also reveal persistent structural barriers affecting both physical and psychological capacities, including budget constraints, high turnover of public officials participating in MICs, logistical challenges in reaching the most vulnerable populations, and limitations in monitoring and information systems. In terms of social opportunity, enduring gender norms, cultural practices, and family-level resistance hinder participation and the effectiveness of preventive actions. These social barriers, along with the perception of excessive bureaucratic burden, negatively affect motivation—particularly among community agents—to engage in and promote intersectoral initiatives. Additionally, participants reported that increasing insecurity and violence in the country reduce direct contact between social services and populations, hindering the implementation of initiatives to combat CCM.

Our study concludes that intersectoral cooperation is a key component in the design and implementation of policies related to sustainable food systems [3]. Strengthening institutional capacities, reducing bureaucratic burden, improving information systems, and promoting gender-sensitive and culturally appropriate approaches are essential actions to enhance coordination and optimize intersectoral responses.

[1] UNICEF (2021). Mesas intersectoriales cantonales para la prevención y reducción de la desnutrición crónica infancia. Guía metodológica para su conformación. Disponible en: https://www.unicef.org/ecuador/sites/unicef.org.ecuador/files/2023-10/Herramienta%204_Guia%20Mesas%20Cantonales.pdf

[2] Michie S, van Stralen MM, West R. The behaviour change wheel: A new method for characterising and designing behaviour change interventions. Implement Sci. diciembre de 2011; 6(1):1-12.

[3] Van der Vliet N, den Broeder L, Romeo-Velilla M, Staatsen B, Kruize H, Friedrich B, et al. Facilitators and barriers of intersectoral co-operation to promote healthier and more environmentally friendly behaviour: a qualitative evaluation through focus groups for the INHERIT project. BMC Public Health. 29 de marzo de 2022; 22(1):617.

# Characterizing the Retail Food Environment in the Barcelona Metropolitan Area


**Letícia Machado**

*Universidade de São Paulo, Brazil*

**Marta Garcia-Sierra**

*FISABIO, Spain*

**Marta Andreu Espuña**

*Institut Metròpoli, Spain*

**Elena Domene Gómez**

*Institut Metròpoli, Spain*


Today, more than half of the world's population lives in urban areas, and it is estimated that approximately 70% of the world's food is consumed in cities, making them key spaces for food systems. Within these systems, the food environment has emerged as a critical component shaping dietary behaviors. The consumer food environment refers to the physical, economic, and social space where people acquire food. In the context of globalization and the industrialization of the food system, the availability of ultra-processed foods has increased, contributing to the deterioration of dietary habits and the rise of non-communicable chronic diseases. In large cities, these dynamics are unevenly distributed across the territory, giving rise to phenomena such as food deserts and food swamps. This study aims to analyze and categorize the retail food environment in the Barcelona Metropolitan Area (AMB) to identify the presence of food swamps, defined as areas with a predominance of outlets offering unhealthy foods. A case study was conducted using secondary data from official bodies and research centers, taking census tracts as the spatial unit of analysis. A total of 14,992 food retail outlets were identified and georeferenced, and classified as healthy, unhealthy, or mixed based on existing literature. To characterize the food environment, the Modified Retail Food Environment Index (mRFEI) was used, applying a spatial analysis with 450-meter buffers from centroids adjusted to residential areas, and assessing three different scenarios depending on the classification of supermarkets and prepared food outlets, with a 0.5 cutoff point to identify food swamps.

The results of the mRFEI show a high prevalence of food swamps in the AMB. In the most permissive scenario, approximately 67% of the analyzed territory was classified as a food swamp, increasing to 83% in the intermediate scenario. In the most restrictive scenario, where supermarkets and prepared food outlets are classified as unhealthy, 93% of the territory is identified as a food swamp. In all scenarios, a significant proportion of areas completely lack healthy food outlets. These findings reveal a widespread presence of unhealthy food environments in the AMB, regardless of the methodology applied. The classification of supermarkets is particularly relevant, given their central role in access to healthy foods, especially outside the city of Barcelona. Although supermarkets have the potential to support healthy diets, their strong promotion of ultra-processed products limits this effect. In conclusion, more than 65% of the AMB presents an unfavorable food environment, highlighting the need for public policies aimed at regulating the retail food supply, promoting healthy outlets, and reducing territorial inequalities in access to adequate food.

# Between Policy and Practice: Evaluating the Financial and Environmental Sustainability of Domestic Agriculture in the UAE

**Eva Vang**

*NYU, Abu Dhabi*

In a country where most of the land is desert, rainfall is scarce, and temperatures remain extreme for much of the year, the prospect of a thriving domestic agricultural sector may appear implausible. Yet the United Arab Emirates (UAE) has made transforming its food system a national priority, not in response to immediate shortages, but in recognition of its long-term vulnerability. With more than 85% of its food imported, the country remains exposed to global supply chain disruptions, price volatility, and geopolitical shocks. To reduce this dependence, the UAE launched its National Food Security Strategy, which aims to produce 50% of its food domestically by 2051 through multi-billion-dollar investments in agricultural technology, subsidies, and farmer support programs. However, the extent to which these top-down initiatives translate into viable, sustainable outcomes at the farm level remains insufficiently examined. This study addresses that gap by asking: How are farmers in Abu Dhabi experiencing and responding to government efforts to strengthen the agricultural sector, and what do their perspectives reveal about the financial and environmental sustainability of food production in the UAE?

This qualitative study draws on eight semi-structured interviews with agricultural stakeholders in Abu Dhabi: seven farm-level actors (CEOs, managers, and agricultural specialists from hydroponic and organic farms) and one food security expert from the Abu Dhabi Agriculture and Food Safety Authority (ADAFSA). Interviews were conducted virtually and lasted 45–60 minutes.

Findings indicate that while the UAE has constructed a robust policy framework to enhance domestic production, structural and environmental constraints limit its contribution to long-term food security. Emirati landowners benefit from subsidies such as free irrigation water, subsidized electricity, and startup financing; however, farms are typically managed by expatriate operators who face bureaucratic barriers in accessing such support, even when formally delegated authority.

Environmental sustainability, central to long-term food security, remains fragile. Although water-efficient technologies such as hydroponics are promoted, high installation costs and inconsistent water quality discourage adoption of this technology. Free water subsidies from the government weaken incentives for conservation, and the absence of groundwater monitoring limits regulatory enforcement. Inadequate agricultural waste management systems result in resource losses, undermining efficiency in a water-scarce environment.

Financial viability also constrains domestic food production. Farmers report high infrastructure costs, revenue declines of up to 70% during extreme summer months, and difficulty competing with low-cost imports in an open market. These pressures threaten farm continuity, limiting the sector's capacity to meaningfully reduce reliance on imports.

Strengthening domestic agriculture is central to the UAE's food security ambitions, yet food security cannot be achieved through production targets alone. It depends on ensuring that farms are structurally supported, environmentally sustainable, and economically viable. The study demonstrates that current policies, while ambitious, require more inclusive implementation mechanisms, stronger water governance, improved waste infrastructure, and enhanced market protections to translate national strategy into resilient food systems. A more farmer-centered and sustainability-driven approach is essential to align domestic agricultural expansion with genuine, long-term food security.

Discussant: **Dr. Michela Accerenzi**, *Fundación ETEA/Universidad Loyola Andalucía*

# Soy Protein-Based Bioplastics as Sustainable Matrices for Controlled Iron Delivery in Horticulture

**Carmen María Granados-Carrera**

*University of Seville, Spain*

**Daniel Castro-Criado**

*University of Seville, Spain*

**Victor M. Perez-Puyana**

*University of Seville, Spain*

**Alberto Romero**

*University of Seville, Spain*

The growing global food demand has intensified agricultural production and the use of fertilizers, which possess low nutrient-use efficiency. Controlled-release fertilizers are sustainable alternatives that allow gradual nutrient delivery synchronized with plant uptake, highlighting bioplastics derived from renewable and biodegradable resources. Soy protein isolate (SPI), a by-product of the soybean oil industry, is a promising candidate for developing nutrient-carrier bioplastics. This study investigates the influence of plasticizers on the physicochemical, mechanical, morphological and functional properties of SPI-based bioplastics and evaluates their performance as controlled-release systems for horticultural applications.

Bioplastic matrices were produced using SPI as polymer, plasticized with water, glycerol, or mixtures (5, 10 and 15 wt%). Iron sulphate heptahydrate (5 wt%) was incorporated as a micronutrient. Tablets were obtained by compression molding (300 bar). The materials were characterized by Fourier transform infrared spectroscopy, thermogravimetric analysis, dynamic mechanical analysis, water uptake capacity (WUC), soluble matter loss (SML), and scanning electron microscopy. Iron release kinetics were evaluated by conductivity. Selected formulations were tested in pepper plants to assess iron bioavailability, plant growth, water consumption and changes in soil properties.

Plasticizer type and concentration had a strong influence on matrix properties. Water-plasticized systems exhibited higher elastic moduli and more compact structures, but lower WUC. In contrast, glycerol increased matrix flexibility, swelling ability and water absorption, although high glycerol content led to increased SML and reduced rigidity. Mixed plasticizer systems showed intermediate behavior and more heterogeneous microstructures. Iron incorporation did not significantly affect thermal stability, but slightly reduced WUC (remaining within suitable ranges for horticulture). Iron release followed a biphasic profile, with an initial rapid release followed by a slower, sustained stage. Systems containing glycerol or mixed plasticizers exhibited more prolonged release, attributed to denser and less permeable microstructures. Crop trials demonstrated that plants fertilized with SPI-based matrices showed increased biomass and leaf number, and improved coloration compared to unfertilized controls, and performance comparable to or better than conventional iron fertilization. Higher iron assimilation was observed in some formulations, confirming their biofortification potential. Additionally, these systems improved soil organic matter and enabled a 30–40% reduction in irrigation water while maintaining adequate soil moisture.

SPI-based bioplastic matrices are effective and sustainable carriers for controlled iron release in horticulture. Plasticizer selection is critical to balance mechanical stability, water absorption and nutrient-release behavior. Overall, these materials enhance crop performance, improve nutrient-use efficiency, reduce water consumption and valorize agro-industrial by-products, supporting circular economy and sustainable agriculture.

**Funding sources:** This research is part of the project with reference SOL2024-31712, cofounded by UE - Ministerio de Hacienda y Función Pública - Fondos Europeos - Junta de Andalucía - Consejería de Universidad, Investigación e Innovación. Authors acknowledge the financial support of Agencia Andaluza de Cooperación Internacional para el Desarrollo through the project "Fortalecimiento de las capacidades de investigación e innovación tecnológica de la UNAH para el desarrollo de cultivos biofortificados mediante el uso de matrices bioplásticas enriquecidas con micronutrientes como fertilizantes sostenibles (Honduras)" (expedient 2025UC005).

# Roadmap for Promoting the Right to Food in Community Gardens

**Felipe Jardim**

*Tilburg University, Netherlands*

Community gardens are urban agriculture spaces that combine physical elements (such as land, composting systems, and gardening tools) and non-physical components (like organized governance, funding, and knowledge sharing). Maintained by volunteers with or without public support for funding, technicians or inputs, these gardens utilize sustainable practices like agroecology to produce food. They offer significant advantages for society (for instance, social inclusion and community sense), the economy (such as household cost reduction and income generation), and the environment (including biodiversity and climate resilience). They are linked to multiple human rights (health, education, freedom of reunion, etc.), with particular relevance to the right to food (food availability, accessibility, acceptability, and sustainability). Based on this context, a qualitative case study was conducted between 2019 and 2023 focusing on community gardens in Berlin, Germany, and Rio de Janeiro, Brazil. Data collection included documents, photographic records, and online and in-person interviews (semi-structured and in-depth) with 40 participants (gardeners, researchers, policymakers, and representatives of gardening groups), 20 in each city. A comparative framework was used, applying thematic analysis to both theory and practice.

Despite their benefits, community gardens face multiple challenges that limit their potential. These include legal and institutional restrictions, such as land tenure insecurity and low political visibility, along with limited access to essential resources like water, funding, and seeds. They are also affected by urban-specific risks such as soil and air pollution, gentrification, and vandalism, as well as organizational barriers like lack of technical knowledge and support networks. To address these issues, it is vital to engage public authorities in establishing formal policies that protect and promote the right to food as part of sustainable local governance. This includes integrating community gardens into urban planning and legal frameworks (e.g., master plans), ensuring land tenure, labour rights, and specialized public management. Recommended strategies involve improving access to resources (water, seeds, knowledge, financing), implementing safety and quality protocols to reduce environmental risks, investing in technical training, and linking community gardens to housing programs to transform idle land into productive spaces. These measures can empower communities and align urban development with sustainability and human rights.

# Agri-food Strategies of the Andean Population to Combat Food Insecurity

**María Nilda Varas Castrillo**

*Universidad Nacional Agraria La Molina, Peru*

In Andean countries, Quechua and Aymara community members continuously create and recreate agri-food strategies to cope with periods of food insecurity caused by climate variability (such as droughts and floods) or socioeconomic crises, drawing on their knowledge and practices in managing the biodiversity within their communal territories. This work is based on an ongoing interdisciplinary research project entitled *"Genomic analysis, genetic and morphological variability of wild potatoes or 'araq papa' associated with polycultures in communities of the Southern Highlands of Peru,"* carried out by researchers from UNALM (Lima), UNSAC (Cusco), and IIES-UNAM (Mexico), and funded by PROCIENCIA (Peru). The study aims to identify the strategies used by Quechua communities to face food insecurity during socio-environmental crises; to document the knowledge and practices related to the production and consumption of araqa papa (wild potatoes) in times of household and community food shortages; and to understand their nutritional value, cultural relevance, and environmental benefits among Quechua populations in Cusco. Information was collected by the Public Nutrition research team on local knowledge and cultural practices associated with agri-food strategies used by Quechua families to cope with climatic and socioeconomic crises, particularly through the use of araqa papas. A qualitative methodology with an ethnographic approach was applied to understand perceptions, meanings, and practices within their social and cultural context. Fieldwork was conducted in two Quechua rural communities during sowing, hilling, and harvesting periods (December 2025 and January 2026), as identified in previous research (Parra et al., 2021), complemented with quantitative data.

Findings show that community members, from a food sovereignty perspective, continue to use agri-food strategies that combine cultivated crops with the consumption of non-domesticated plants. Crop diversity in family plots for self-consumption plays a key role in ensuring food security. During times of crisis, communities rely on ancestral knowledge and practices related to local wild flora and fauna to secure food, thereby preserving a rich reservoir of local agrobiodiversity and ensuring community-level food self-sufficiency. The research conducted so far confirms the ongoing adaptation and recreation of agri-food strategies by Quechua farmers who operate in environments characterized by high climatic variability and uncertainty. These communities anticipate yearly agricultural conditions based on natural indicators and signals. Within this communal and family planning—especially in adverse agricultural years—they turn to araqa papa, referred to as the "mother potato," as a key alternative to alleviate hunger. In other years, its consumption becomes a staple when food reserves are depleted or diminished, highlighting its central role in sustaining food systems and resilience.

# Bridging Food Policy and Practice: Policy-operational Translation Capacity in Agrifood Systems

**Canberk Genc**

*Rural PM Academy, Spain*

Food policies increasingly aim to enhance resilience, sustainability and food security across agrifood systems. However, implementation outcomes remain uneven across territories and value chains. While regulatory frameworks and strategic objectives are often well articulated, their translation into coordinated daily practice frequently encounters structural bottlenecks. This study investigates recurring implementation patterns across diverse agrifood contexts and examines how coordination routines, decision structures and learning mechanisms influence the materialization of policy intentions. The objective is to identify operational conditions that shape the effectiveness and continuity of food policy interventions.

A qualitative multi-case study was conducted across primary producers, food processors, food service operators and policy-supported territorial initiatives operating within sustainability and innovation frameworks. Data were collected through structured system-mapping workshops, organizational diagnostics, field observation and facilitated coordination sessions. Pre and post-intervention reflective assessments documented changes in decision clarity and coordination practices. Cross-case synthesis was applied to identify recurring bottlenecks independent of sector or scale. Analytical clustering focused on patterns of decision latency, responsibility allocation, communication structures and feedback mechanisms influencing implementation continuity.

Five recurrent implementation bottlenecks emerged consistently across cases: (1) decision latency in multi-actor governance environments; (2) fragmented responsibility structures generating duplication or execution gaps; (3) absence of structured learning loops linking pilot activities to routine practice; (4) misalignment between policy time horizons and operational cycles; and (5) coordinator overload caused by fragmented communication flows. These bottlenecks were associated with delayed implementation of sustainability measures, reduced adaptive capacity under climatic or market variability, limited institutionalization of pilot outcomes and youth disengagement linked to administrative burden and unclear roles. In contexts where structured coordination routines and short reflection cycles were introduced, qualitative improvements were observed in role clarity, reduction of recurring friction, shorter problem-resolution cycles and stronger alignment among territorial actors. Learning retention shifted from episodic to cumulative, supporting greater operational continuity.

Findings indicate that food policy effectiveness is conditioned not only by regulatory design and financial instruments but also by policy-operational translation capacity within agrifood systems. Strengthening coordination routines, clarifying responsibilities and embedding structured feedback mechanisms may enhance resilience and food security outcomes by improving implementation stability and adaptive capacity. The study contributes an applied analytical framework for understanding how operational environments mediate policy materialization across diverse agrifood contexts. Future research may extend this analysis through longitudinal and quantitative evaluation of translation capacity indicators.

# Why Poultry Farmers Leave the Industry: An Investigative Study from Middle East: The Case of Iraq

**Sanar Muhyaddin**

*Wrexham University, United Kingdom*

While global demand for poultry and poultry products continues to rise, the number of poultry farms in Iraq has declined by 34% over the past five years. This study examines the wide range of factors influencing poultry farmers' decisions to exit the industry prematurely. Although these factors have been identified across diverse individual studies, there remains a lack of comprehensive understanding regarding which factors are most influential and how they interact within a single contextual framework. To address this gap, the study adopts an explanatory sequential mixed-methods design, beginning with a questionnaire survey (n = 450), followed by in-depth interviews (n = 21) with both current and former poultry farmers in Iraq.

The findings from this research will contribute to the literature on agribusiness survival in hostile business environments and its implications for food security. The mixed methods approach also highlights key areas for future research. Furthermore, the study sheds light on the challenges faced by poultry farmers and the strategies they use to survive in a complex, unstable environment. It offers practical recommendations for policymakers and international stakeholders to better target interventions to improve the resilience and performance of the poultry sector in Iraq.

Discussant: **Dr. Ana Paula Lamoso**, *Universidad Pablo de Olavide*

# Mind the Agriculture-Health-Gap: Aligning European Food Supply with National Dietary Guidelines and Planetary Health Diet

**Anna-Lena Klapp**

*University of Göttingen, Germany*

**Josh Bisig**

*ProVeg International, Germany*

**Daniel Braune**

*ProVeg International, Germany*

**Joanna Trewern**

*ProVeg International, Germany*

National food-based dietary guidelines (FBDGs) are essential policy instruments designed to bridge nutritional science and public health. However, adherence remains low across Europe, where diets are characterized by excessive animal source food intake and insufficient consumption of legumes and vegetables. Because food environments are shaped in part by production, trade, and subsidies, it's critical to assess whether agricultural and trade systems actually supply food in alignment with dietary recommendations. Furthermore, the healthfulness of diets is inseparable from environmental sustainability; current global food systems are primary drivers of climate change and biodiversity loss. This study aims to quantify the inconsistencies between current food supply and dietary recommendations. Specifically, we compare national FBDG recommendations and the Planetary Health

Diet (PHD) reference diet to actual agricultural production and food supply for 34 European countries.

We conducted a dietary gap analysis for 34 European countries with FBDGs published as of December 2025. Data on national food supply and agricultural production were sourced from FAO Food Balance Sheets. FBDG recommendations were standardized into 11 food groups and harmonized with FAO commodity categories using a methodology adapted from Springmann et al. (2020). Food supply and self-sufficiency were calculated for three scenarios: current consumption, FBDG-aligned consumption, and PHD-aligned consumption. To ensure comparability, per-capita recommendations were adjusted for food loss to calculate the total supply required for population-level adherence. Data processing was performed using Python for cleaning, conversion, and statistical analysis.

Preliminary results reveal a systemic oversupply of animal products and a chronic undersupply of plant-based foods. Red meat oversupply is the most extreme: approximately 94% of countries provide more red meat than recommended, with a median oversupply factor of 3.7x. Notably, Spain's supply is nearly 13 times its national recommendation. Conversely, 80% of European countries fail to meet vegetable supply targets, and 76% face deficits in legumes. At the aggregate European level, the red meat supply stands at 393% of FBDG-aligned requirements, while legumes (61%) and vegetables (63%) show significant deficits. Regarding self-sufficiency, only 15% of countries produce enough vegetables to meet their own FBDG requirements. When measured against the Planetary Health Diet (PHD), the aggregate European red meat supply reaches 615% of recommended levels, while legumes (8.7%) and vegetables (74%) show profound deficits. This demonstrates a stark structural misalignment between current agricultural production and nutritional goals, necessitating a heavy reliance on imports to address the shortage of nutrient-dense plant crops.

A massive agriculture-health-gap exists in Europe, where agricultural specialization—driven by historical and economic priorities—directly contradicts public health and environmental goals. Overall, European food systems disproportionately favor food groups that should be limited while failing to adequately supply those recommended for healthy, sustainable diets. This is a missed opportunity to enable needed dietary shifts and requires a fundamental realignment of agricultural production and trade policies. Bridging this gap is essential for building a resilient food system that supports both human and planetary health.

# The Milan Pact in Latin America: Urban Food Governance in Bogotá and Mexico City

**Cristian Murcia**

*Universidad de Valencia/Universidad Nacional de Colombia, Spain/Colombia*

The Milan Urban Food Policy Pact serves as a global framework guiding governments toward sustainable food systems through six strategic areas: governance; sustainable diets and nutrition; social and economic equity; food production; supply and distribution; and food waste reduction. In Latin America—one of the regions with the highest number of signatory cities—the Pact is particularly relevant in urban contexts characterized by deep social inequalities, high levels of economic informality, and persistent tensions between market forces, the state, and territory. This study critically analyzes the implementation of the Milan Pact in Latin America from a political economy perspective, using Bogotá and Mexico City as case studies. It examines how the Pact's strategic areas are adopted and reinterpreted in practice through power relations, institutional arrangements, and economic dynamics that shape urban food systems. A qualitative comparative approach was employed, including documentary analysis of public policies, urban development plans, food strategies, and regulatory frameworks implemented in both cities following their adherence to the Pact. This was complemented by a critical review of academic literature on food policy, urban governance, and the right to food. The six Pact areas were used as analytical categories to assess the degree of institutionalization, intersectoral coherence, and transformative capacity of urban food policies, considering both their formal progress and structural limitations.

The findings show that in both cities the Milan Pact has been incorporated selectively. Progress has been made in the governance area through the creation of coordination and participation spaces; however, these mechanisms have limited influence on structural decision-making within urban food systems. Regarding sustainable diets, Bogotá and Mexico City have strengthened public food programs and nutrition education, which nonetheless coexist with food environments dominated by agro-industrial products and ultra-processed foods. In terms of social and economic equity, persistent tensions remain—although vulnerable populations are recognized as policy targets, the right-to-food approach is only partially operationalized and largely through assistance-based measures. In the areas of production, supply, and distribution, advances include local procurement initiatives and proximity markets, but these have limited capacity to challenge power structures concentrated in large intermediaries. Food waste management appears as the least integrated area within urban planning. Overall, the Milan Pact has functioned primarily as a normative and discursive framework rather than a tool for structural transformation. Its implementation highlights the limitations of urban food policies when underlying power relations are not addressed. Advancing toward sustainable cities in Latin America requires politicizing the Pact's principles, embedding them more firmly in urban planning, strengthening a rights-based approach to food, and confronting market dynamics that perpetuate food inequality.

# The Informed Consumer Paradox: Soft Claims and Parental Vulnerability to Food Marketing

**María de los Ángeles López Amián**

*Universidad Loyola Andalucía, Spain*

**Alazne Arraztio**

*Universidad Loyola Andalucía, Spain*

**María José Montero Simo**

*Universidad Loyola Andalucía, Spain*

Food packaging targeted at children constitutes a key persuasive tool in purchase and consumption decisions within the household (Hallez et al., 2020). Through food marketing, packaging can highlight positive attributes that do not always reflect the actual nutritional quality of products, thereby influencing purchasing choices. In this context, Soft Claims—unregulated statements such as "natural," "homemade," or "traditional"—have significantly increased their presence in foods aimed at children, despite not necessarily being associated with healthier nutritional profiles (López et al., 2016; Arraztio-Cordoba et al., 2023). In a context of rising childhood obesity, current regulations prioritize the protection of children, giving less attention to the role of parents as purchasing agents and mediators in these decisions. This study examines how Soft Claims on children's food packaging influence food choices, considering both children and the role of parents as mediators or barriers to these marketing strategies. The research consisted of two complementary experimental studies conducted in Spain with 128 children and 89 parents. Data were collected through Qualtrics using a standardized visual experiment in which participants viewed images of identical foods that differed only in the presence or absence of Soft Claims, allowing their isolated effect to be assessed. Stimuli were presented individually and sequentially on mobile devices, within schools for children and remotely for parents, ensuring comparability of results through the use of the same procedure and platform.

The results show that Soft Claims increase product preference in both groups, with a much stronger effect observed among parents. Among children, products with Soft Claims obtained a mean score of 6.61 (SD = 1.54) compared to 5.39 (SD = 1.54) without claims ($t = 6.32$, $p < 0.001$, $d = 0.79$). Among parents, the difference was even more pronounced: 11.56 (SD = 1.22) with Soft Claims versus 5.10 (SD = 1.0) without them ($t = 38.55$, $p < 0.001$, $d = 5.78$). These findings challenge the notion of adults as fully rational decision-makers and as effective barriers against food marketing strategies targeting children. Rather than counteracting the influence of packaging, parents appear highly sensitive to Soft Claims, showing stronger persuasive effects than children. This highlights the capacity of such strategies to shape consumption decisions even among groups traditionally considered more informed. Overall, the results suggest that regulatory approaches focused exclusively on children may be insufficient to address the commercial determinants of childhood obesity. The study underscores the need for more integrated regulatory frameworks that recognize packaging as a persuasive tool directed at both children and adults, thereby supporting the development of public policies aligned with the Sustainable Development Goals and the promotion of healthier and more socially responsible diets.

# Drivers of Food Security in Morocco: A Dynamic Analysis of Multidimensional Determinants

**Berrak Nada**

*Cadi Ayyad University, Morocco*

**El khider Abdelkader**

*Cadi Ayyad University, Morocco*

Food security is a multi-domain concept that remains difficult to operationalize within a single analytical framework. Although it constitutes a central pillar of economic development and population well-being, food security does not necessarily depend on domestic food production or caloric availability. In many developing contexts, it results from the interaction of economic, social, productive, institutional, and environmental factors. A key challenge in the literature concerns both the measurement of food security and the identification of its dominant determinants. Most empirical studies rely on partial indicators or pre-computed indices, often neglecting agency and sustainability dimensions. The study therefore aims to identify the key drivers of food security in Morocco by adopting a block-wise econometric strategy and constructing an original composite index integrating six dimensions: availability, access, utilization, stability, agency, and sustainability.

The analysis focuses on Morocco over the period 2000–2023, using data from FAOSTAT, the World Bank (WDI), the World Governance Indicators, and WHO. A composite Food Security Index (FSI) is constructed following OECD (2008) guidelines using a nested structure approach. To identify determinants, a block-wise econometric strategy is adopted to avoid over-parameterization in a small-sample context. Ordinary Least Squares (OLS) estimations serve as a benchmark, while Autoregressive Distributed Lag (ARDL) models capture short-run, delayed, and long run dynamics. The blocks include economic factors (income, inflation, food imports), social and demographic factors (unemployment, education, urbanization), production and environmental variables (food production, agricultural value added, arable land, $CO_2$ emissions), as well as institutional and financial mediators.

Robustness is ensured through unit root tests, bounds tests for cointegration, diagnostic checks, stability tests (CUSUM), and Toda–Yamamoto causality tests.

The composite index reveals a two-phase trajectory of food security in Morocco, with sustained improvement between 2000 and 2020 followed by a sharp decline after 2021, reflecting heightened vulnerability to inflationary pressures and external shocks. Index decomposition shows that the utilization dimension, reflecting investments in water, sanitation, and health infrastructure, while access and stability remain structurally fragile, mainly drove past improvements. Econometric results indicate that income growth and food imports improve food security only in the short run, whereas inflation exerts a strong negative effect with delayed and causal impacts. Unemployment significantly undermines food security in both the short and long run, while urbanization displays non-linear dynamic effects. By contrast, food production, agricultural value added, and environmental variables do not exhibit robust long-run relationships with food security. Institutional quality and agricultural credit do not emerge as significant dynamic mediators.

The findings reveal a structural paradox: Morocco has strengthened food utilization capabilities yet remains constrained by persistent weaknesses in economic access and stability. These results challenge production-centered narratives and strongly support Sen's entitlement approach, showing that food insecurity is driven less by food availability than by purchasing power erosion and labor market conditions. The absence of long-run effects from productive variables underscores the limits of output-centered strategies and highlights the importance of inflation control, employment, and access-oriented policies.

Discussant: **Dr. Alfonso Sánchez-Carrasco,** *Universidad Pablo de Olavide*

# Food Transition as Climate Policy: Public Procurement and Family Farming for Resilient Food Systems

**Adriana C. Torres Bastidas**

*Dejusticia, Colombia*

The paper seeks to analyze public food procurement regulation as a strategic climate adaptation instrument within the framework of Nationally Determined Contributions (NDCs) under the Paris Agreement. For this purpose, it examines how procurement frameworks linked to food systems particularly school feeding and social protection programs—can operationalize NDC commitments related to adaptation, food security, and resilient agriculture. Additionally, the document aims to assess, in the Colombian context, the extent to which public procurement regulation supports food transition and strengthens climate resilience, while identifying structural barriers that limit its effectiveness in current NDC implementation.

The study adopts a qualitative research design combining regulatory and policy analysis with a case study approach. Data collection includes a systematic review of Colombia's NDCs, climate adaptation policies, and food system–related strategies, alongside an in-depth analysis of public procurement regulations and school feeding program rules. The analysis is complemented by semi-structured interviews with peasant and family farmers, public procurement officials, local authorities, and program implementers, as well as field-level observations of procurement processes and food supply chains. Data were analyzed thematically using an integrated food systems, climate adaptation, and rights-based analytical framework.

Preliminary analysis shows that food systems and agriculture are priority areas for climate adaptation. However, this recognition is only weakly translated into public procurement regulation. Evidence from the Colombian case reveals three categories of barriers that undermine the participation of family and peasant farmers in school feeding programs: formal barriers, reflected in regulatory frameworks that establish documentary requirements—such as tax registration and sanitary certifications—that are of difficult or impossible compliance for rural populations with limited connectivity and institutional support; material barriers, particularly the absence of timely payment mechanisms, since smallholders without access to credit cannot sustain participation in public markets that pay thirty or more days after delivery; and structural barriers, rooted in the historical conditions of discrimination and exclusion facing the peasantry, including restricted land size, lack of mechanization, limited associativity, and poor access to credit and infrastructure.

The study adds to the discussion about how procurement regulation that allows for preferential access for family farmers, flexible contracting mechanisms, and territorial sourcing can function as a concrete adaptation measure aligned with NDC objectives. Such regulatory designs contribute to diversified production systems, stabilize rural incomes, reduce vulnerability to climate shocks, and enhance the resilience of food supply for public programs. In contrast, rigid procurement frameworks, administrative complexity, and reliance on intermediaries undermine the contribution of procurement to NDC implementation and weaken food system resilience. The analysis suggests that rather than treating procurement as a secondary or technical instrument, climate policy frameworks should recognize it as a structural lever for food systems transformation—one that requires regulatory coherence across climate, agricultural, and social protection policies to ensure that NDC commitments move beyond declarative targets toward operational implementation.

# Innovation for Rural Communities in Mozambique: Remote Sensing for Agroclimatic Stress Identification and Decision-Making Toward Precision Family Farming

**Guillermo Palacios-Rodríguez**

*University of Córdoba, Spain*

**David Ariza-Mateos**

*University of Córdoba, Spain*

**Vanesa Domínguez-Bermúdez**

*University of Córdoba, Spain*

**David Martínez-Meléndez**

*CESAL, Spain*

**Carolina Santos-Portillo**

*University of Córdoba, Spain*

**Mª Ángeles Varo-Martínez**

*University of Córdoba, Spain*

Agriculture in southern Mozambique is highly exposed to extreme climate events, particularly droughts and floods, which recurrently compromise agricultural production. This vulnerability is further intensified by limited availability of up-to-date climate information, a reduced capacity to identify early signs of crop stress, and the lack of operational information and technical advisory systems that support near–real-time decision-making by farmers in rural areas. In response to this scenario, the University of Córdoba (UCO) has promoted in recent years the development of various technological solutions aimed at strengthening the resilience of rural communities in Mozambique by generating and forecasting agroclimatic information to improve technical advisory processes and optimize agricultural management. Within two interventions funded by the Andalusian Agency for International Development Cooperation (AACID), implemented in partnership with the Provincial Directorates of Agriculture of Gaza and Maputo and the NGO Bosque y Comunidad, an initial remote crop stress detection tool was designed and implemented based on the Google Earth Engine cloud computing platform.

This tool takes the form of a visual and interactive web application available in Portuguese, integrating data from Sentinel-2 and MODIS satellite imagery. Based on these data, several spectral vegetation indices are calculated for complementary purposes: NDVI to estimate vegetation vigor and growth; NDMI to assess plant water content; MSI as an indicator of water stress; NDWI to detect variations in surface water presence; and SIPI to identify potential physiological changes related to pests or diseases. In a later phase, building on lessons learned, the University of Córdoba significantly optimized the tool within an intervention funded by the Spanish Agency for International Development Cooperation (AECID) and led by the NGO CESAL. This improved version expands operational functionality by incorporating climate forecasting into the decision-making framework, using an alternative index (VHI) that combines NDVI and land surface temperature, increasing analytical specificity through crop-specific thresholds, and enhancing the dynamic nature of results by aligning them with different crop phenological stages. These advancements contribute to moving family farming toward precision agriculture models adapted to the Mozambican rural context.

# Holistic Livestock Management for the Restoration of Desertified Lands in the Sahel


**Pasquier Hélène**

*Action Against Hunger, Spain*

**Cadario Joaquin**

*Action Against Hunger, Spain*

**Gueye Mama**

*Action Against Hunger, Senegal*


According to estimates by the United Nations Convention to Combat Desertification, 45% of the Earth's land surface is affected by land loss, impacting 3.2 billion people [1]. In the Sahel, widespread desertification and soil degradation are contributing to the decline of natural resources and land productivity, undermining the livelihoods of populations highly dependent on agriculture and livestock, and reducing their resilience to climate change.

One of the main factors contributing to desertification is the overgrazing of vegetation (grasslands, shrubs, trees) due to conventional livestock management. Since 2024, Action Against Hunger has been working with pastoralist communities in the Déaly silvopastoral reserve in northern Senegal, using the Holistic Management (HM) approach. HM promotes the restoration of degraded environments by considering the interrelationship between environmental, economic and social factors. Community-based grazing planning, one of the key tools of HM, facilitates the planned movement of herds, ensuring, on the one hand, good nutrition for the livestock and, on the other, sufficient rest time for the recovery of pastures. Short, intensive grazing cycles, followed by long rest periods, help improve the water cycle, soil nutrient cycles, biodiversity and biomass production. In just two years of intervention (2024 and 2025), Action Against Hunger has observed improvements in the experimental field: vegetation cover has increased from 0% (completely bare soil) in July 2024 to 50% by the end of the 2025 dry season, and to over 70% on average in October 2025, at the end of the rainy season. No signs of wind erosion are now observed across the entire surface of the experimental field, and sheet water erosion is detected only at a few isolated points. Biomass production, estimated using visual methods with local herders, has increased by 60% from 2024 to 2025, although an invasive species of low forage value, endemic to the entire region, persists. Finally, more than two months after the last rains, satellite imagery (Sentinel-2 SWIR images from 31/12/2025) shows higher soil moisture within the field compared to the surrounding areas.

This pilot project aims to provide the pastoralist communities of Déaly with a methodology to help them improve the management of their resources, thereby strengthening their livelihoods. The results obtained so far have generated interest in increasing the area under HM and in replicating the project in other pastoral areas of Senegal.

[1] UNCCD. (2024) "Global Land Outlook Thematic Report on Rangelands and Pastoralism. United Nations Convention to Combat Desertification," Bonn.

# Psychosocial Determinants of Solastalgia Among Colombian Indigenous Communities in Contexts of Polycrisis

**Marcela Guapacha Montoya**

*Universidad de Manizales, Colombia*

**Felipe Agudelo Hernández**

*Universidad de Manizales, Colombia*

**Valentina González Carreño**

*Universidad de Manizales, Colombia*

**Andrés Camilo Delgado Reyes**

*Universidad de Manizales, Colombia*

The objective of this study was to examine the association between psychosocial factors—including resilience, hopelessness, substance use, family problems, adverse childhood experiences, and food insecurity—and solastalgia in two Colombian Indigenous communities (Embera Dobidá people) living in contexts of polycrisis. The study hypothesized that factors such as resilience, hopelessness, problematic substance use, family difficulties, adverse childhood events, and structural conditions such as displacement or food insecurity may help explain solastalgia in Embera Dobidá communities. A cross-sectional design was implemented in two Indigenous communities in Chocó as part of a broader public mental health intervention program. Participants (n = 142, aged 7 to 21 years) completed validated instruments, including the Connor-Davidson Resilience Scale, the Brief Solastalgia Scale (a five-item Likert-type scale assessing demographics, health, life satisfaction, climate-related emotions, and connection with nature, translated and validated in Colombia among Embera Dobidá communities), the CRAFFT screening tool for adolescent substance use risk, the PACES scale (measuring parenting, behavior, emotions, and suicide risk), and the Food Security Scale. Correlation and multiple regression analyses were performed.

Solastalgia was significantly associated with hopelessness, resilience, and food insecurity, with the regression model explaining 55.8% of the variance in solastalgia scores. Hopelessness emerged as the strongest predictor ($\beta = .521$, $p < .001$), followed by resilience, family problems, substance use, and food insecurity. Bivariate correlations further showed that solastalgia was significantly associated with age, hopelessness, food insecurity, and adverse childhood experiences. These findings provide empirical evidence on the psychosocial determinants of solastalgia among Embera Dobidá youth in Chocó, Colombia, highlighting the central role of hopelessness and food insecurity, while suggesting that individual resilience may exert a complex and potentially risk-aware protective effect. Future research should be led by Indigenous communities, adopt longitudinal designs to track solastalgia across developmental stages and changing environmental conditions, and integrate objective environmental indicators (e.g., mercury levels, deforestation rates) with psychosocial measures. Additionally, research should explore how these findings can be integrated with traditional Indigenous healing frameworks to develop culturally appropriate interventions.

# Vulnerability to Food Poverty in Spain: Insights from the Spanish Household Budget Surveys (2006–2024)

**Victor Martinez-Cano**

*Basque Centre for Climate Change, Spain*

**Chiara De Tomassi**

*Basque Centre for Climate Change, Spain*

**Manuel Tomás**

*Basque Centre for Climate Change, Spain*

**Iñaki Arto**

*Basque Centre for Climate Change, Spain*

**Iker Etxano**

*Basque Centre for Climate Change, Spain*

**María José Sanz**

*Basque Centre for Climate Change, Spain*

**Inma Batalla**

*Basque Centre for Climate Change, Spain*

Agrifood systems are major contributors to climate change and other ecological pressures, while simultaneously being affected by environmental degradation and failing to ensure access to healthy and nutritious diets for all. Food security is eroded by both shocks and structural stresses. Recent disruptive events—including the Covid-19 pandemic, the war in Ukraine, and increasingly frequent climate extremes—have exposed underlying vulnerabilities that hinder these systems from guaranteeing food security, particularly for vulnerable populations. As a result, food insecurity has gained increasing attention, also in the Global North and the EU. Food insecurity is shaped by diverse interconnected and overlapped factors that belong to different dimensions. However, in these contexts, food insecurity is primarily related to limited access to healthy and nutritious food due to insufficient purchasing power. Although various studies have explored food insecurity in the EU using quantitative and qualitative approaches, official measurements remain scarce. In Spain, only one study has addressed food insecurity measurement to date (Moragues-Faus & Magaña-González, 2022). This work aims to bridge this gap by using Spanish Household Budget Surveys (HBS) to assess economic vulnerability in access to healthy and sustainable diets over the period 2006–2024.

Food poverty among Spanish households is assessed using four food poverty lines (FPLs) estimated through two approaches. The first is based on a relative "at risk of food poverty" (AROFP) indicator. The remaining three are derived from the estimated annual cost of dietary guidelines considered healthy and sustainable: the Mediterranean Diet, the Planetary Health Diet, and the Spanish Dietary Guidelines. Households with food expenditure below these FPLs, adjusted by equivalent consumption units, are classified as vulnerable. Household food expenditure is estimated using HBS microdata, while FPLs are calculated using regionalized food price data from the Spanish Consumption Panel of the Ministry of Agriculture, Fisheries and Food (MAPA).

The share of households vulnerable to food poverty increased between 4.43% and 6.68% from 2006 to 2024, depending on the indicator used. In 2024, 24.91% of Spanish households were classified as vulnerable according to the AROFP indicator, while estimates based on dietary cost ranged from 13.90% to 19.71%. Significant territorial and social disparities are observed. Increases in food poverty have been more pronounced in urban and peri-urban areas and among specific household types, including large families, single-parent households (particularly single-mother households), and non-standard household configurations. In relative terms, food expenditure shares show a trend towards equalization between lower- and higher-income households, especially since 2020.

These findings align with existing literature and current trends but highlight the limitations of quantitative food poverty indicators, which depend on threshold definitions that require validation through complementary qualitative approaches.

Future research should also consider interactions between food expenditure and other essential costs such as housing, energy, and transport. This study provides a quantitative basis for assessing vulnerability to food insecurity and contributes to advancing food insecurity measurement in Spain.

Discussant: **Dr. Tomás Palmisano,** *Universidad de Buenos Aires*

# Bioplastic Matrices from AgroWaste for Controlled Iron Delivery in Sustainable Horticulture

**Carmen María Granados-Carrera**

*Universidad de Sevilla, Spain*

**Daniel Castro-Criado**

*Universidad de Sevilla, Spain*

**Víctor Manuel Pérez Puyana**

*Universidad de Sevilla, Spain*

**Alberto Romero García**

*Universidad de Sevilla, Spain*

The need to increase food production while minimizing environmental impacts has intensified the search for more efficient fertilization strategies. Conventional fertilizers often show low nutrient-use efficiency, leading to soil degradation, nutrient losses, and higher irrigation demands. In parallel, large amounts of agro-industrial residues remain underutilized despite their potential as renewable feedstocks for biodegradable materials. This study develops bioplastic matrices using protein- and starch-rich agro-waste—soy protein and pea protein isolates, and cassava starch—as controlled-release carriers for iron in horticultural systems. The objectives are to assess (i) how polymer composition and plasticizer type affect the physicochemical, mechanical, thermal, and morphological properties of the matrices; (ii) their iron-release behavior in soil and aqueous media; and (iii) their agronomic performance regarding plant growth, nutrient assimilation, soil quality, and water-use efficiency.

Bioplastic matrices were produced by compression molding using soy protein, pea protein or cassava starch. Water, glycerol, and mixed plasticizers were added at different concentrations to adjust flexibility, water interaction and microstructure. Iron sulfate heptahydrate was incorporated as micronutrient. Materials were characterized by FTIR, TGA, dynamic mechanical analysis, water uptake and SEM. Iron release was evaluated in aqueous media and soil. Greenhouse trials with pepper plants assessed iron bioavailability, biomass, leaf development, soil organic matter, and irrigation needs.

Protein-based matrices showed higher mechanical stability and more compact structures than starch-based systems. Water-plasticized materials were more rigid, while glycerol increased flexibility, swelling, and permeability. Mixed plasticizers produced intermediate viscoelastic behavior and heterogeneous microstructures. Iron incorporation preserved thermal stability and only slightly altered water-related properties. Iron release followed a biphasic pattern, with an initial rapid phase followed by a sustained release. Glycerol-containing and mixed-plasticizer matrices enabled more prolonged release due to reduced permeability and denser internal structures. Soil assays confirmed controlled nutrient delivery over several weeks. Greenhouse trials showed increased biomass, improved leaf development, and enhanced coloration compared with unfertilized controls. Iron assimilation matched or exceeded conventional fertilization, and the matrices contributed to higher soil organic matter and reduced irrigation requirements while maintaining adequate moisture.

Agrowaste-derived bioplastics offer a promising strategy for sustainable horticulture by improving nutrient-use efficiency, enhancing soil health, and valorizing agricultural residues. Plasticizer selection is a key factor influencing mechanical stability, water interaction, and nutrient-release behavior. Agronomic results indicate that these materials can match or exceed conventional fertilization while supporting water conservation and soil regeneration. Overall, this approach aligns with circular-economy principles and provides a scalable pathway to strengthen food-system resilience and crop nutritional quality.

Funding sources: This research is part of the project with reference SOL2024-31712, cofounded by UE - Ministerio de Hacienda y Función Pública - Fondos Europeos - Junta de Andalucía - Consejería de Universidad, Investigación e Innovación. Authors acknowledge the financial support of Agencia Andaluza de Cooperación Internacional para el Desarrollo through the project "Fortalecimiento de las capacidades de investigación e innovación tecnológica de la UNAH para el desarrollo de cultivos biofortificados mediante el uso de matrices bioplásticas enriquecidas con micronutrientes como fertilizantes sostenibles (Honduras)" (expediente 2025UC005).

# Tradition as Innovation: Heritage-led Food Production

**Juan-José Raposo-González**

*Independent Researcher, Spain*

Since the final third of the 20th century, agro-industrial paradigms have expanded globally, prioritizing profitability through intensive mechanization and chemical inputs. While this model has increased yields to sustain a burgeoning global population, it has simultaneously precipitated ecological degradation, the erosion of genetic resources, and the economic marginalization of small-scale farmers. Although modern technological innovation seeks to mitigate this global crisis, a fundamental question arises: should we not first look to traditional ecological knowledge? This study aims to reassert the pertinence of traditional practices held by rural communities, positioning them as essential frameworks for addressing climate challenges and contemporary environmental ethics.

Across diverse disciplines, there is an increasing academic recognition of traditional practices as viable alternatives to productivist models. This research identifies the core values that position traditional agricultural systems as blueprints for the future through a systematic review of theoretical and practical discourses within the United Nations framework. The methodology involves an analysis of key international charters regarding heritage, the environment and sustainable development, alongside an examination of the designations for traditional agricultural landscapes established primarily by UNESCO and the FAO.

The findings demonstrate that the environmental consciousness of traditional societies is intrinsically woven into their ancestral practices. The sustainable stewardship of agricultural resources constitutes a form of living heritage that bridges the natural, cultural, and intangible spheres. These complex systems comprise a multifaceted array of elements, including indigenous seed varieties, specialized cultivation techniques, and sophisticated water management strategies. Historically, this vernacular knowledge has been transmitted orally through rituals, myths, and folklore. While some practices have been scientifically validated and integrated into modern "organic farming" or "permaculture" frameworks, this appreciation often depends on external scientific legitimacy, which frequently fails to acknowledge the cultural origins and communal ownership of such knowledge.

Traditional agricultural practices are indispensable for addressing the modern imperative of sustainable, community-oriented, and climate-resilient food production. However, much of this intangible heritage remains undervalued and is currently at risk of disappearance. Furthermore, the tension between maximizing short-term productivity and preserving long-term natural resources remains a central debate. While traditional systems may not match the sheer output of agro-industrial models, their centuries-long persistence provides empirical evidence of their resilience and long-term viability in the face of fluctuating climatic and social conditions.

# Bioactive-Rich Colombian Fruits as Supporters of Sustainable Diets and Food Security

**Juan Carlos Carmona-Hernández**

*Universidad de Manizales, Colombia*

Tropical and Amazonian fruits represent an underutilized resource for strengthening sustainable food systems, particularly in biodiverse countries such as Colombia. Beyond their nutritional value, these fruits are rich in polyphenols and flavonoids—bioactive compounds with antioxidant and anti-inflammatory properties that can contribute to improved dietary quality. Vastly recommended beneficial foods include olive oil, nuts, and avocado (Mediterranean diet); for many Latin-American communities these items are expensive. Multiple varieties of fruit grow in Tropical areas; different climates, geographical conditions, and water resources favor their cultivation and harvesting. Several passion fruits are economically important in Colombia. *Mauritia flexuosa* (aguaje) and *Theobroma grandiflorum* (copoazú) are distributed in the Amazon region, in Colombia, Venezuela, the Guyanas, Trinidad, Ecuador, Peru, Brazil, and Bolivia. These Colombian fruits report applications, not only for food, but also for medical purposes considering edible and non-edible components. This study aims to synthesize scientific evidence on selected Colombian and Amazonian fruits and to analyze their potential contribution to sustainable food systems, food security, and health-oriented food policies.

Bioactive compounds (polyphenols and flavonoids) were extracted from edible and non-edible parts of Colombian fruits. A comparative analysis of different studies was conducted focusing on the polyphenolic composition, antioxidant capacity, and biological activity of fruits *Passiflora ligularis, Passiflora popenovii, Mauritia flexuosa* (aguaje/buriti), and *Theobroma grandiflorum* (copazu). Total polyphenol and flavonoid content, biochemical assays, antioxidant stability tests, and bioactivity indicators were examined to assess both nutritional functionality and potential applications within sustainable food and health systems.

Different laboratory tests demonstrated that these fruits (edible and non-edible parts) contain high levels of polyphenols and flavonoids with significant antioxidant, anti-inflammatory, antiglycemic, and lipid peroxidation–inhibiting activities. Extracts from *Mauritia flexuosa* and *Theobroma grandiflorum* showed notable radical scavenging capacity, while *Passiflora* species exhibited effective anti-inflammatory activity and stable antioxidant activity over extended storage periods. The flavonoid-to-polyphenol ratios were found to influence antioxidant efficacy, highlighting the functional value of biodiversity-based food sources. These characteristics position tropical fruits as nutritionally dense foods with potential for value-added products and health-promoting diets.

The findings underscore the relevance of tropical and Amazonian fruits as strategic components of sustainable and resilient food systems. Their high bioactive content supports not only improved nutrition and public health but also diversification of agricultural production and local food systems—key factors for food security in the context of climate change and socio-economic vulnerability. Integrating these fruits into food policies, agri-food value chains, and dietary guidelines can contribute to sustainability, rural development, and the right to adequate food. This evidence supports the need for interdisciplinary approaches linking agricultural science, nutrition, and food policy to fully harness biodiversity for equitable and sustainable food futures supporting, initially multiple rural families and transcending to urban areas.

# Governing Dietary Norms for Sustainable Consumption: A Comparative Analysis of Policy Instruments in China and the EU

**Yi Lu**

*Peking University, China*

Dietary norms—socially constructed expectations of what constitutes healthy or desirable eating—are increasingly recognized as a critical lever for sustainable food system transformation. Yet the regulatory mechanisms through which states reshape these norms remain under-explored in comparative legal scholarship. China and the European Union represent two distinct paradigms: China has shifted from moral exhortation to quasi-legal enforcement through the Anti-Food Waste Law (2021) and the "Clean Your Plate" campaign, while the EU pursues multi-layered governance anchored in the Farm to Fork Strategy (2020) and front-of-pack labeling initiatives such as Nutri-Score. This study comparatively analyzes how both jurisdictions deploy soft law, economic instruments, and supply chain standards to govern dietary norms, identifying which configurations demonstrate greater institutional resilience in steering sustainable consumption.

A comparative institutional analysis framework is applied across three dimensions: (1) soft law and nudging—mapping China's 32-article Anti-Food Waste Law and its penalty regime against the EU's voluntary Nutri-Score system adopted in seven member states; (2) economic instruments—comparing China's Soybean Rejuvenation Plan and Three-Year Action Plan for Reducing Soybean Meal in Feed (2023) with the EU's Common Agricultural Policy (CAP) 2023–2027 Eco-scheme allocations and 25% organic farming target; (3) supply chain standards—assessing green certification frameworks including the EU–China Geographical Indications Agreement. Data sources comprise primary legislation, official policy documents, and peer-reviewed empirical studies. Outcomes are evaluated through quantitative indicators, including food waste reduction rates, subsidy-induced planting area changes, and organic farmland expansion.

The analysis reveals divergent institutional logics with mixed effectiveness. On the soft law dimension, China's shift from moral to legal governance produced measurable but uneven outcomes: pilot restaurant programs achieved approximately 20% food waste reduction, yet the nationwide loss rate remains at 22.7% (460 million tons annually), indicating enforcement gaps. In the EU, Nutri-Score expanded to nearly 1,000 registered companies with 1,420 brands following the 2024 algorithm update, but political resistance from states such as Italy and the absence of mandatory harmonization have fragmented its normative impact. On economic instruments, China's soybean subsidies yielded a 23.22% increase in sown area, and the 2023 feed-reduction initiative cut soybean demand by over 9 million tons. EU organic farmland grew from 5.9% (2012) to 10.8% (2023), though the pace must more than double to reach the 25% target by 2030. On supply chain standards, the EU–China Geographical Indications Agreement established mutual recognition for over 200 products, creating a bilateral framework defining "qualified" food through provenance-based norms.

China's top-down, sanction-reinforced model achieves rapid normative signaling but encounters compliance deficits at the local level, while the EU's polycentric approach offers broader stakeholder engagement at the cost of slower harmonization. Neither model alone demonstrates sufficient resilience for governing dietary norm transitions at scale. Effective governance requires a hybrid regulatory architecture combining mandatory behavioral standards with market incentives and supply chain certification. These findings contribute to understanding how general norms in food systems can be institutionally reconstructed, offering implications for building more resilient food governance frameworks.

# A Healthy, Dignified, and Sustainable Food Base: Development and Validation of Basic Food Baskets for Populations at Risk of Food Insecurity in Spain

**Sara Tulipani**

*Action Against Hunger, Spain*

**Yael Puyol-Martín**

*Universitat Ramon Llull, Spain*

**Beatriz Tamayo-Borrajo**

*Action Against Hunger, Spain*

**Pablo Soriano-Jofre**

*Action Against Hunger, Spain*

**Antonio Vargas-Brizuela**

*Action Against Hunger, Spain*

**Elena Carrillo-Álvarez**

*Universitat Ramon Llull, Spain*

Action Against Hunger's Healthy Eating and Lifestyles strategy seeks to address, through an intersectoral approach, the structural barriers and social determinants of food insecurity that hinder conscious, healthy, equitable, and sustainable food choices, particularly among people experiencing poverty and socioeconomic exclusion. The cost of a healthy diet is one of the main structural determinants to be addressed. In addition, current food systems exert significant pressure on the environment—including contributions to greenhouse gas emissions—highlighting the need to promote healthy and sustainable diets adapted to all socioeconomic groups. The aim of this study was to develop, monetize, and validate, through a participatory, inclusive, and multicultural approach, Basic Food Baskets adapted to different territorial contexts in Spain.

The methodological design follows the Reference Budget approach (Carrillo-Álvarez 2016, 2021) and is structured in five phases: (1) Definition of the study scope, including the identification of relevant socioeconomic profiles, the construction of reference individuals across life-cycle stages, and the selection of regions representative of Atlantic and Mediterranean dietary patterns, with rural/urban stratification; (2) Basket construction and pricing, translating dietary and sustainability recommendations (AESAN 2022; EAT-Lancet 2025) into specific food lists, classified according to sustainability levels based on seasonality, packaging, and point of purchase; (3) Participatory validation, through the implementation of four mixed focus groups per territory (rural/urban; adult/adolescent, n = 8–10) to assess social and multicultural acceptability and practical feasibility; (4) Pricing in affordable retail outlets and inclusion of basic kitchen equipment; and (5) Adjustment and knowledge transfer.

The study demonstrates the feasibility of operationalizing basic food baskets that simultaneously integrate health, environmental sustainability, and economic affordability criteria, adapted to different territories and socioeconomic contexts in Spain. The Reference Budget approach makes it possible to identify how the gradual incorporation of sustainability criteria—such as seasonality, local sourcing, and minimal packaging—has differentiated effects on the final basket cost and its alignment with diverse dietary practices.

Participatory validation provides key insights for food policy decision-making by highlighting practical barriers and structural constraints affecting the adoption of healthy and sustainable diets among vulnerable populations, particularly regarding price, available time, and cooking skills. Overall, the monetization of healthy and sustainable baskets offers an operational tool to guide social benefits, food assistance programs, and food education strategies that are sensitive to territorial context and cultural diversity.

## References


Carrillo-Álvarez et al. *Public Health Nutrition*. 2016, 19(17): 3232–3244. doi:10.1017/S1368980016001026

Carrillo-Álvarez et al. *Sustainability*. 2021, 13(16), 9401; https://doi.org/10.3390/su13169401

Spanish Agency for Food Safety and Nutrition (AESAN). 2022, *Scientific Committee Journal,* ISSN 1885-6586, 36, 11–70.

Rockström et al. The EAT–Lancet Commission on healthy, sustainable, and just food systems. *The Lancet,* Volume 406, Issue 10512, 1625–1700.

Discussant: **Dr. Alfonso Sánchez-Carrasco,** *Universidad Pablo de Olavide*

# Participation of Colombian Indigenous Adolescents for Food Insecurity After Migration

**Felipe Agudelo Hernández**

*Universidad de Manizales, Colombia*

**Marcela Guapacha Montoya**

*University of Caldas, Colombia*

**Juan Carlos Carmona**

*Universidad de Manizales, Colombia*

Adolescents from Indigenous communities more frequently experience multiple crises. Migration due to armed conflict makes it necessary to explore cultural strengthening and adolescent participation in community recovery mechanisms. This study explored, within a Colombian Indigenous population, the potential associations between wellbeing and health participation, and the variables affected during processes of polycrisis and migration. It also analyzed the actions undertaken by adolescents in their communities to address psychosocial suffering.

This study adopted a longitudinal, explanatory and longitudinal design, conducted at three points in time after migration. The quantitative component involved designing an instrument to determine the participation of Indigenous adolescents in health. Validated instruments were also used to determine mental health problems, environmental suffering, food security, health problems, and aspects related to migration. Regression models were used for exploratory purposes, and the three measurement points were compared, with post-hoc analyses.

A significant improvement trend was identified in variables related to participation and general well-being, with statistically significant differences (<.001) among the three measurement points. The final model for the first measurement point accounted for 79.8% of the variance (adjusted $R^2 = .798$). Model stability was supported by VIF values between 1.357 and 1.55, and tolerances between .737 and .645, ruling out multicollinearity issues. Geographic dispersion, limited access to meat, eggs, and milk, and solastalgia were the factors that showed possible association, with a statistically significant difference (<.001). The final model for the second measurement point accounted for 45.4% of the variance (adjusted $R^2 = .454$). The model's stability was supported by VIF values between 1.072 and 1.813, and tolerances between .552 and .933, also without multicollinearity issues. Variables such as geographic dispersion, food insecurity, lack of shelter, and feeling like you were in a foreign culture showed a possible statistically significant association (<.001). At the third time point, the model contributed 44.5% of the variance (adjusted $R^2 = 0.445$), with a Durbin-Watson statistic of 1.839. VIF values between .961 and .974 and tolerances between 1.027 and 1.04 were found. At this time point, although geographic dispersion and food insecurity persisted as possible associated factors, adolescent participation emerged as a factor with a possible relationship to spiritual disharmony.

This study proposes an integrated understanding of the well-being of Indigenous adolescents in contexts of forced displacement in Colombia, one that transcends approaches focused exclusively on improving material conditions or individual health indicators. It reveals that post-displacement adjustment processes are profoundly mediated by cultural, spiritual, and community dimensions, as well as by the active role of adolescence in social reconfiguration. By highlighting solastalgia and migration grief as culturally situated phenomena, the study expands the literature on Indigenous mental health by incorporating analytical categories sensitive to the connection with territory. This study suggests that adolescent participation could act as an articulating axis between health, spirituality, and community reconstruction in contexts of forced displacement, underscoring the need for intercultural approaches that recognize Indigenous adolescents not only as an affected population but also as active agents of care, decision-making, and social transformation.

# The Making of the Right to Food: Tracing Food Policy Conflict and Trade-offs in Colombia

**Felipe Roa-Clavijo**

*Universidad de los Andes, Colombia*

This paper traces how food policy debates evolved inside Colombia's peace process between the National Government and FARC-EP and how they later shaped implementation. It asks how negotiators moved from an early clash between food sovereignty and food security toward a shared settlement around the right to food, and what political trade-offs that shift implied for policy design. A qualitative document analysis approach was utilized, and process tracing was applied to reconstruct negotiation sequences across exploration (2012), negotiation (2012–2016), and implementation (2017 onwards). An analytic sample was constructed from official repositories and formal civil society forum reports. Findings were triangulated through interviews with former negotiators and through cross checking with research on parallel negotiations between the National Government and agrarian movements.

The analysis identifies four stages. First, food sovereignty was advanced by FARC-EP as a rights-based challenge to the prevailing economic model, while a food security framework was defended by the National Government and trade policy and sovereignty claims were excluded from the agenda. Second, food sovereignty was placed on hold, and disagreement was managed through relabeling toward food and nutrition and hunger eradication language, while a partial rural reform agreement was reached. Third, the right to food was adopted by both parties as an overarching framework, including a plan for progressive realization that aimed to restructure institutions and address hunger and malnutrition. Fourth, right to food framing was sustained during implementation, but participation varied, with strong territorial engagement through development programs with a territorial approach (PDET) design alongside more technocratic national policy process.

The paper shows that a discussion that began as a peace negotiation generated major and lasting shifts in Colombia's food policy field. The peace accord trajectory contributed to the adoption of the right to food as a constitutional right and embedded right to food commitments within the National Development Plan 2022 to 2026. By doing so, the peace process opened space for policy change and reframed long standing disputes that had remained politically blocked for decades, moving them into formal state agendas and institutional design debates.

# Food Security as an Instrument of Oeacebuilding: The Contributions of Food Security Policies to Lasting Peace

**Irene Jiménez-Zumalde**

*University of the Basque Country, Spain*

**Karlos Pérez de Armiño**

*University of the Basque Country, Spain*

According to Jonas Galtung, peacebuilding refers to the activities that "remove the causes of war and offer alternatives to war in situations where war might occur." This broad definition has resulted in different proposals about what constitutes peacebuilding that change depending on the view of peace followed. In this paper, I understand peacebuilding as a long-term process that has the following characteristics: aims at positive peace, deals with the core causes of conflict, transforms structures and power dynamics of society confronts gender inequalities at all levels, enforces local participation and local agency, and considers cultural diversity.

In this sense, food security policies contribute to such peacebuilding processes as they fulfil the previously mentioned characteristics: Food security projects have been able to improve livelihoods, which has contributed to social cohesion, reconciliation and enforces the local resilience capabilities that improve the answers to shocks. These projects are not limited to the short-term needs, and they contribute to the social wellbeing, reduction of vulnerabilities, and promotion of a more sustainable use of resources. The projects that answer the needs of the population and improve the inclusion of marginalized groups implemented by authorities, improve the confidence in them. As a result, the power relations between the different social groups will transform into a more equal one.

The communities are the ones that better known their needs and the best ways to respond to them, which shows the need to include the community. At the same time, local food systems and livelihoods are essential in the peacebuilding process to reduce the marginalization of certain social groups. The food security projects go beyond the nutritional aspect because they involve changes in education and health sectors. Those changes are essential to create social security networks which will create diverse ways to achieve peace. Gender lenses have shown that women are more vulnerable to food insecurity due to the gender power imbalances in the access to land, and land property rights that harm women's ability to the food secure. Therefore, food security projects that deal with issues of land use and property can reduce the gender inequalities. The projects of food security can happen at any time, they are suitable to prevent conflict, they can reduce the negative impacts of violence in the population, and they present ways to reconstruct societies after the conflict. Therefore, they are long-term projects that are not limited to the post-conflict contexts.

In short, food policies that go beyond meeting short-term food needs and succeed in promoting alternative livelihood systems for the population, they as well as improve local governance, reduce inequalities within communities, and address the root causes of conflict, which are essential for peacebuilding. The goal of this paper is to present which kind of food policies contribute to the previously described peacebuilding processes and which do not.

# Anticipating Hunger in Conflict Settings: Data-Driven Approaches to Support Humanitarian Action, Food Policy and IHL in Fragile Contexts

**Julien Jacob**

*Action Against Hunger, Spain*

**Hélène Pasquier**

*Action Against Hunger, Spain*

**Jorge Hernández Marín**

*University of Granada, Spain*

**Ronny Meza Acosta**

*University of Granada, Spain*

**Francisco Javier Abarca Álvarez**

*University of Granada, Spain*

Hunger affects nearly 700 million people worldwide and is disproportionately concentrated in regions affected by armed conflict. Conflict-driven displacement, disruption of food systems, and restrictions on humanitarian access increasingly intersect with climate shocks and economic instability, intensifying food insecurity and household vulnerability. Effective realignment of food security policies therefore requires analytical approaches that capture the mechanisms through which conflict drives food insecurity and inform timely, evidence-based humanitarian and policy responses.

This paper builds on the MEFIC (Monitoring and Evaluation of Food Insecurity in Conflicts) methodology, developed by Action Against Hunger Spain and the Hegoa Institute at the University of the Basque Country. MEFIC provides a structured analytical framework to assess how armed conflict affects the three pillars of food security by identifying conflict-related and contextual indicators for availability, access, and utilization. Based on the MEFIC framework, collected information is organized around a set of predefined indicators, with particular attention to violent acts affecting food systems and civilian food security—including attacks, destruction, contamination, and theft—which supports the development of analytical hypotheses linking violent events to food security outcomes.

To enhance visibility, accessibility, and operational use of MEFIC, a digital platform has been developed in collaboration with GIS4tech, a spin-off company from the University of Granada. The platform integrates georeferenced conflict-event data with food security indicators and contextual variables at the municipal level, enabling users to explore spatial and temporal interactions between conflict dynamics and food security outcomes. The platform improves situational awareness in complex emergencies, highlights critical data gaps, and supports humanitarian analysis where direct field assessments are limited.

Building on this data infrastructure, a predictive modeling component based on machine learning has been incorporated. The model uses CatBoost, a gradient-boosted decision tree ensemble, to forecast key food security indicators: the Food Consumption Score (FCS), Household Dietary Diversity Score (HDDS), and reduced Coping Strategies Index (rCSI). Leveraging agroclimatic, socioeconomic, and conflict-related data structured through the MEFIC framework, the model captures complex nonlinear relationships and improves the anticipation of food insecurity trends in conflict settings.

The integration of the MEFIC methodology, the digital platform, and predictive analytics offers significant value for food security policy and humanitarian action. By strengthening early warning and anticipatory analysis, the framework supports more timely and targeted interventions, improved prioritization of humanitarian resources, and enhanced protection of civilian food systems in line with International Humanitarian Law. More broadly, it demonstrates how data-driven approaches can support policy realignment by connecting conflict analysis, food system monitoring, and operational decision-making in fragile contexts.

# FRUGALL PROJECT

**Fertilizing Rural-Urban Grids through Agroecology Living Labs to enhance sustainable food system transitions**

**(03/2026 to 02/2029)**

## 5 Living Labs across different levels of maturity

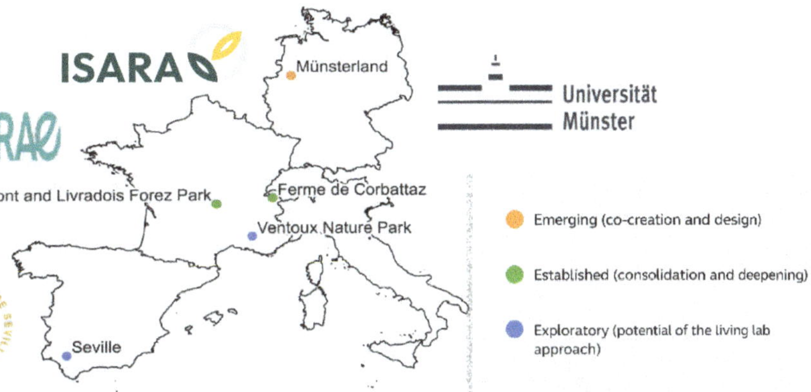


ISARA

INRAE

Universität Münster

## 6 objectives for strengthening rural-urban exchanges for agroecological transition

OBJECTIVE 1

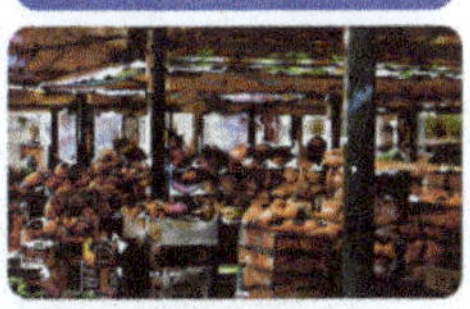

***Regional food system mapping***

Understanding and supporting stakeholder needs.

OBJECTIVE 2

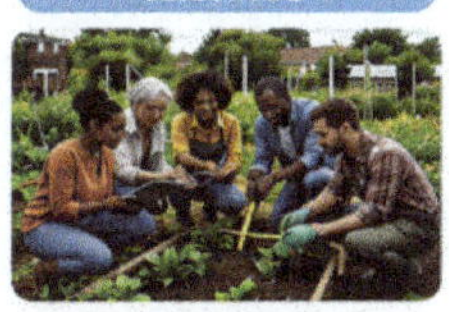

***Agroecology Living Labs***

Co-creating Regional Transition Pathways

OBJECTIVE 3

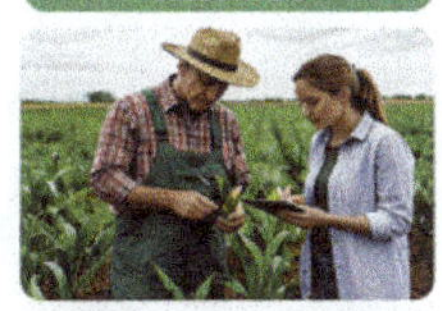

***Piloting Agroecological Innovation***

Working out the Specifications

OBJECTIVE 4

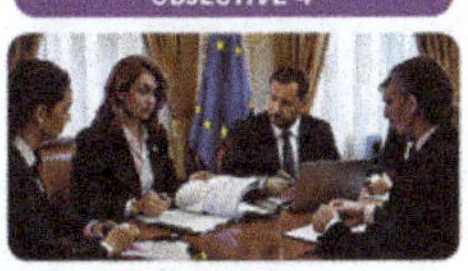

***Risk Assessment I***

Understanding policy barriers and enablers.

OBJECTIVE 5

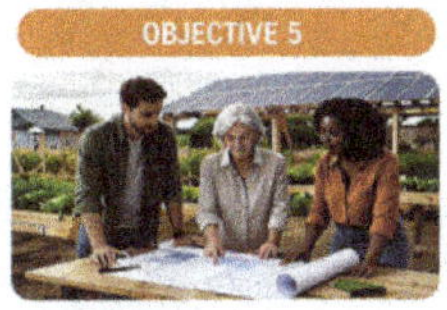

***Risk Assessment II***

Securing Sustainable Impact.

OBJECTIVE 6

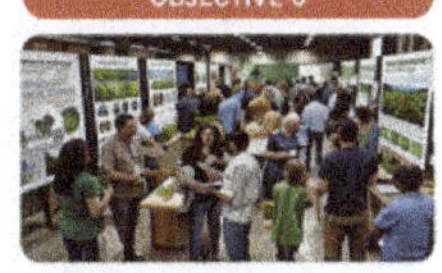

***Communication & Outreach***

Regional Stakeholders Citizens/Consumers

2nd AGROECOLOGY co-funded call
Proyectos de Colaboración Internacional PCI2026-1
Coordination: University of Münster (UoM)
Spanish partner: University of Seville (US)
PI contact at US: mbmarin@us.es

**Scan here and stay updated**

Living Labs, Agroecological innovations, opportunities for cooperation...and much more!

Ulysseus EUROPEAN UNIVERSITY
GOBIERNO DE ESPAÑA MINISTERIO DE CIENCIA, INNOVACIÓN Y UNIVERSIDADES
AGENCIA ESTATAL DE INVESTIGACIÓN
Funded by the European Union
AGROECOLOGY PARTNERSHIP

# Related Titles from Westphalia Press

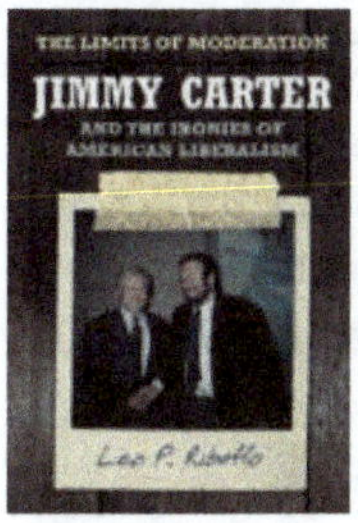


The Limits of Moderation: Jimmy Carter and the Ironies of American Liberalism
by Leo P. Ribuffo

The Limits of Moderation is not a finished product. And yet, even in this unfinished stage, this book is a close and careful history of a short yet transformative period in American political history, when big changes were afoot.

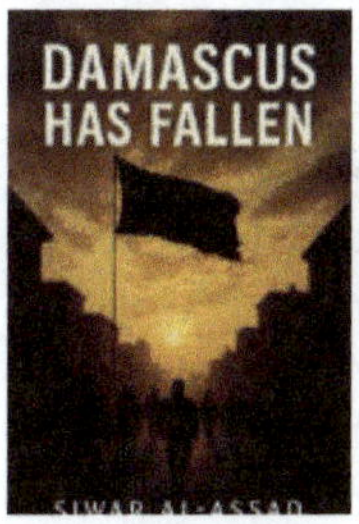


Damascus Has Fallen
by Siwar Al-Assad

In Damascus Has Fallen, we see Syria through the eyes of its storm-tossed people in a place where every place is a secret, every choice a moral quandary and by the minute everything in a person's life can change.

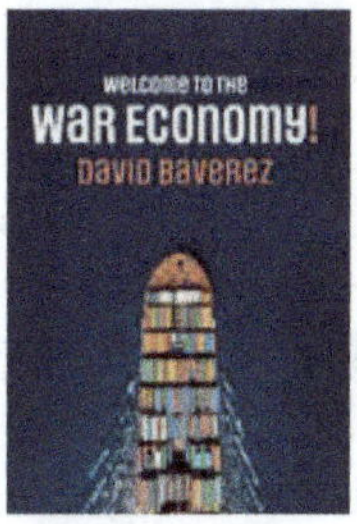


Welcome to the War Economy!
by David Baverez

David Baverez calls for a collective awareness of the changing international balance of power. And at a time when companies are having to contend with profound shifts in value, he suggests measures they can take to rapidly deal with chaos and ensure their survival.

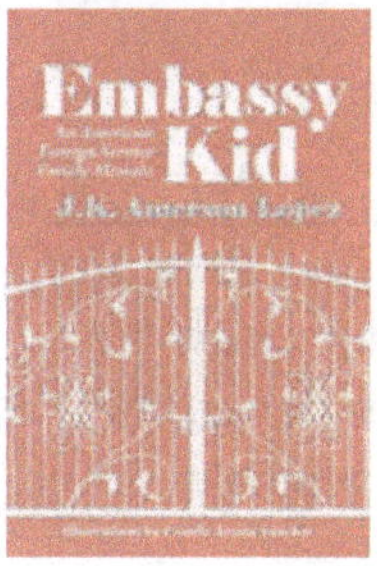


Embassy Kid: An American Foreign Service Family Memoir
by J.K. Amerson López, Illustrated by Camila Acosta Sánchez

Embassy Kid follows Robert and Nancy Amerson, a courageous couple from the American Heartland, and their two daughters as they carry out the mission of the US Information Agency to "win hearts and minds for democracy" in Latin America and Europe during the Cold War.

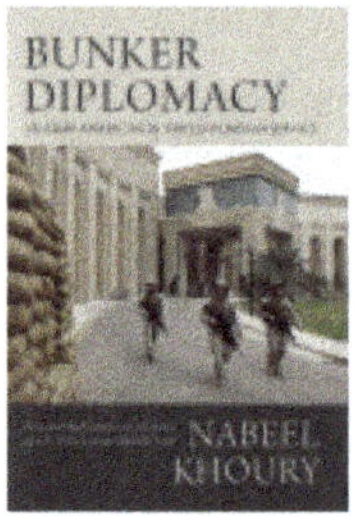


## Bunker Diplomacy: An Arab-American in the U.S. Foreign Service
by Nabeel Khoury

After twenty-five years in the Foreign Service, Dr. Nabeel A. Khoury retired from the U.S. Department of State in 2013 with the rank of Minister Counselor. In his last overseas posting, Khoury served as deputy chief of mission at the U.S. embassy in Yemen (2004-2007).

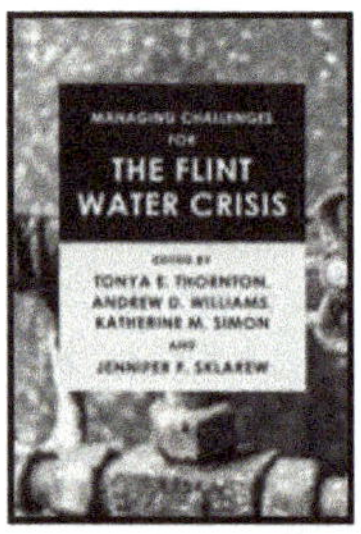


## Managing Challenges for the Flint Water Crisis
Edited by Toyna E. Thornton, Andrew D. Williams, Katherine M. Simon, Jennifer F. Sklarew

This edited volume examines several public management and intergovernmental failures, with particular attention on social, political, and financial impacts. Understanding disaster meaning, even causality, is essential to the problem-solving process.

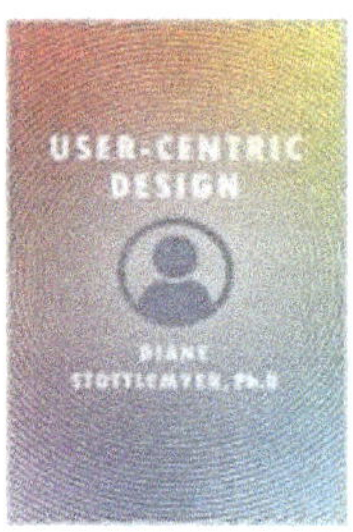


## User-Centric Design
by Dr. Diane Stottlemyer

User-centric strategy can improve by using tools to manage performance using specific techniques. User-centric design is based on and centered around the users. They are an essential part of the design process and should have a say in what they want and need from the application based on behavior and performance.

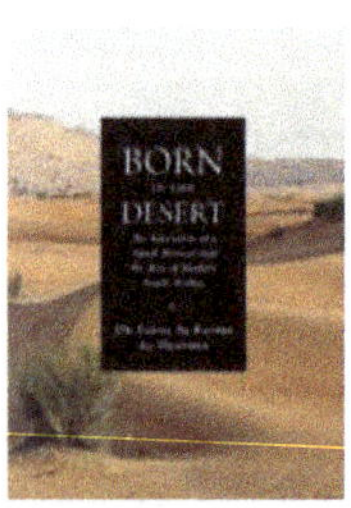


## Born in the Desert: The Education of a Saudi Nomad and the Rise of Modern Saudi Arabia
by Dr. Faisal Al-Mershed

The remarkable story of Dr. Faisal Al-Mershed who was born a Bedouin to an illiterate family and rose to prominence, His life parallels the rise of Saudi Arabia from an underdeveloped, nomadic kingdom to one of the largest and most dynamic economies in the world today.

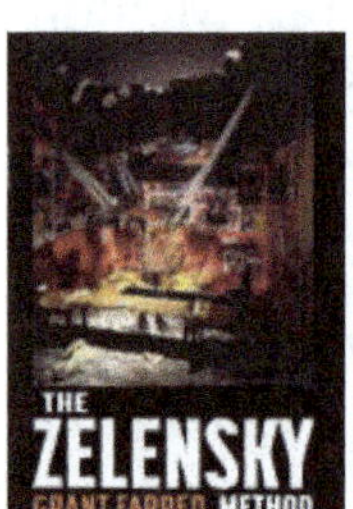


## The Zelensky Method
by Grant Farred

Locating Russian's war within a global context, The Zelensky Method is unsparing in its critique of those nations, who have refused to condemn Russia's invasion and are doing everything they can to prevent economic sanctions from being imposed on the Kremlin.

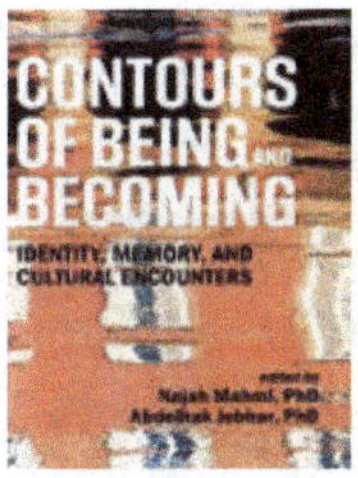


Contours of Being and Becoming: Identity, Memory, and Cultural Encounters
Editors: Najah Mahmi PhD and Abdelhak Jebbar

This project stems from an urgent need to question the human condition within the actual sites of interconnections and divisions, creating glocal bridges and borders.

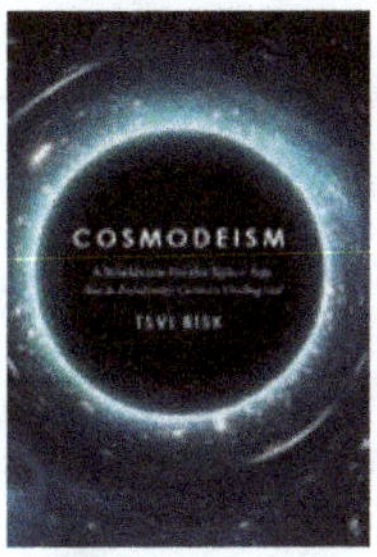


Cosmodeism: A Worldview for the Space-Age: How an Evolutionary Cosmos is Creating God
by Tsvi Bisk

Bisk suggests that understanding our place in this cosmic 'godding' process will go a long way in assuaging that sense of meaninglessness of it all that is the cause of so much civilizational pessimism and angst.

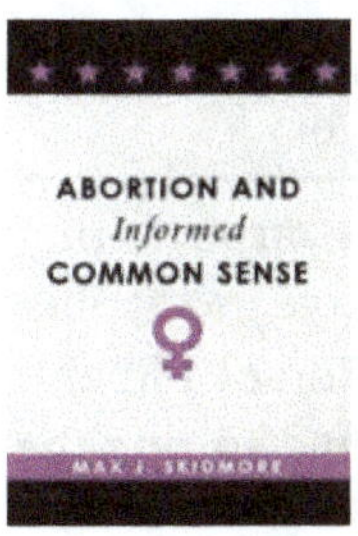


Abortion and Informed Common Sense
by Max J. Skidmore

The controversy over a woman's "right to choose," as opposed to the numerous "rights" that abortion opponents decide should be assumed to exist for "unborn children," has always struck me as incomplete. Two missing elements of the argument seems obvious, yet they remain almost completely overlooked.

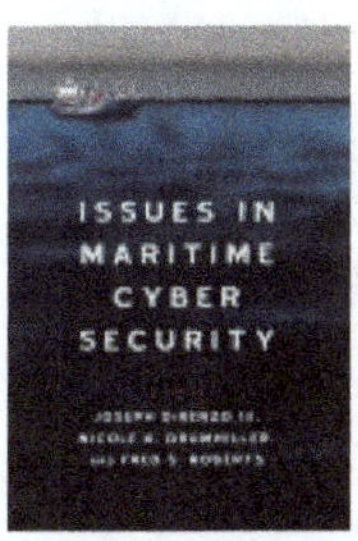


Issues in Maritime Cyber Security
Edited by Dr. Joe DiRenzo III, Dr. Nicole K. Drumhiller, and Dr. Fred S. Roberts

The complexity of making MTS safe from cyber attack is daunting and the need for all stakeholders in both government (at all levels) and private industry to be involved in cyber security is more significant than ever as the use of the MTS continues to grow.

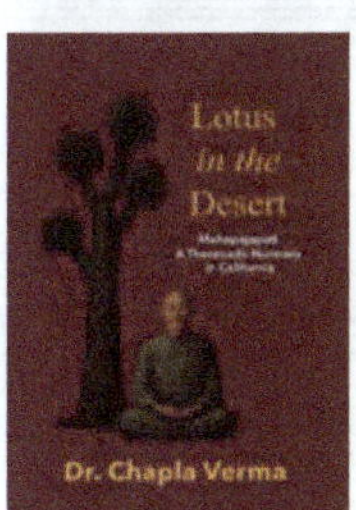


Lotus in the Desert
Mahapajapati: A Theravada Nunnery in California
by Dr. Chapla Verma

This book tells the story of Mahapajapati nunnery and the challenges nuns face to survive as female Theravada Buddhist monastics. The narrative includes the life stories of nuns. Each nun's narrative is just as valid as another's but presents a different perspective.

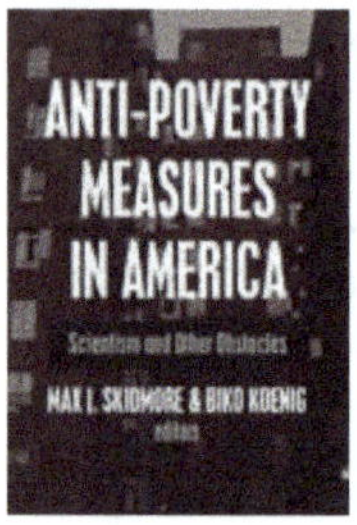


Anti-Poverty Measures in America: Scientism and Other Obstacles
Editors, Max J. Skidmore and Biko Koenig

Anti-Poverty Measures in America brings together a remarkable collection of essays dealing with the inhibiting effects of scientism, an over-dependence on scientific methodology that is prevalent in the social sciences, and other obstacles to anti-poverty legislation.

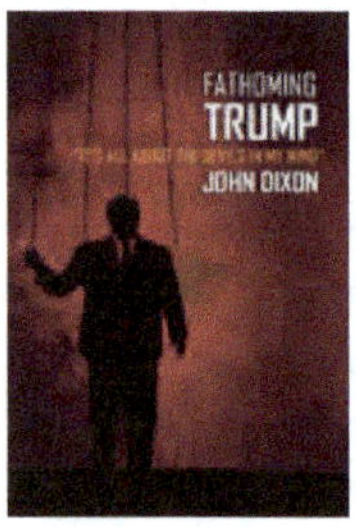


Fathoming Trump: "It's All About the Devils in My Mind"
by John Dixon

This is a very distinctive type of book. It draws upon reporting in the American and foreign media on Trump in business and in politics. It uses explanatory frameworks to explicate his character flaws, his worldview, and his way of thinking.

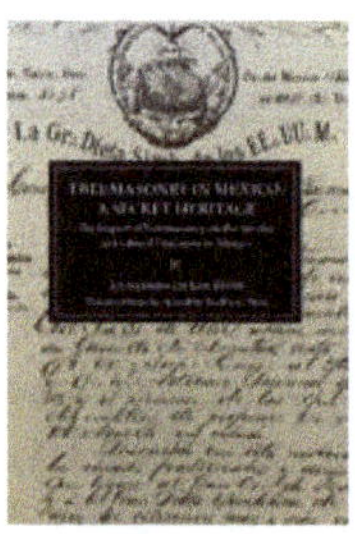

Freemasonry in Mexico: A Secret Heritage
The Impact of Freemasonry on the Secular and Liberal Discourse in Mexico by Guillermo De Los Reyes

In this thought-provoking book, De Los Reyes argues that Freemasonry, through its lodges, played a decisive role in shaping Mexico's national thought, contributing to the creation of a liberal and secular State and fostering anticlerical sentiments among the laity that endured well into the twentieth century.

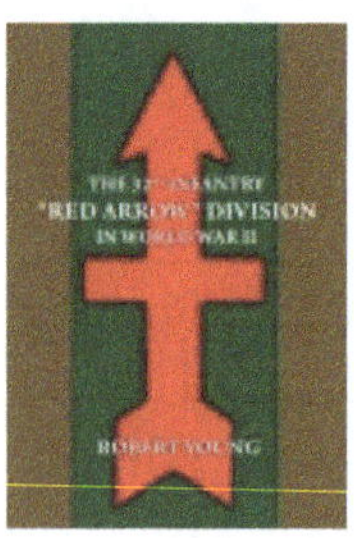

The 32nd Infantry "Red Arrow" Division in World War II
by Dr. Robert Young

If one were to think of famous U.S. Army divisions of World War II, the 32nd Infantry Division would most likely not even be mentioned. Yet, it was the 32nd Infantry Division that spent 654 total days in combat, more than any American unit of the war.

westphaliapress.org

www.ingramcontent.com/pod-product-compliance
Lightning Source LLC
LaVergne TN
LVHW060041210926
848481LV00013B/3925
*9781637235515*